Hand Book of Hair Oils

What Natural Oils Can Do For Your Hair

Lyse Lauren
Ever Here Now Publishing

Preface

I bet you had no idea there are so many different and wonderful oils that can do great things for our hair!

The West has ignored the use of hair oils in recent decades, although their use was very much part of life in days of yore. Now, these oils are receiving more attention and there has been something of a surge of interest in recent years. However, Middle Eastern, Asian and many, many other cultures across the planet have used them for countless decades without interruption.

Hair Oil is the work-horse of Hair Care Products. If there is any one thing that crosses cultures, creeds, countries, and ethnicities, it is Hair Oil. As you read on, you will see that this statement is not an exaggeration.

Why is Hair Oil so important for our hair?

The short answer for that is that hair oils offer multiple benefits for, not only hair but also the skin and scalp. These benefits act interdependently.

The longer answer would have to include at least a few examples of why, and some of the reasons are;

1. It moisturizes and conditions the hair.

2. It helps to heal scalp problems, clear up infections and prevent many of them from occurring in the first place.

3. It makes it easy to brush the hair without breaking and further splitting or damaging the hair ends.

4. It greatly assists in nourishing the hair, replacing vital nutrients that the body is unable to provide naturally.

5. It adds shine and lustre to the hair, enhancing its natural colours.

6. Helps to prevent premature greying.

7. Can stimulate the hair follicles promoting hair growth and regrowth.

8. Protects from harsh environmental conditions such as the wind, heat, and cold.

9. Many hair oils are emollients.

10. Protects against environmental pollutants and the list just goes on and on...

The fact is that it is a cornerstone product for the hair, one that really works and the best part of all of this is that it does this work *naturally*. These are mostly herbal and organic-based oils and the ones we like to promote are cold-pressed and will not have any chemical additives.

We will investigate the many kinds of hair oils available on the market today, what their different strengths and weaknesses are and from this selection of comprehensive articles you should easily be able to choose which oil is just right for you and your hair needs.

Everyone has different hair. Some have thick, some curly, some long, some are losing hair, some are greying prematurely, some have split ends, to name just a few of the problems we might face. We can and should have a basic idea of what problems may exist with our own particular hair type and this book will help you to discover which oil will be the most helpful to you in dealing with whatever hair vulnerabilities you may have.

Even if you just want increased shine and lustre for your hair, this is where you will find out which oil is right for you and why.

The *Handbook of Hair Oils* was created in order to offer a one-stop information spot for all things 'Hair Oil'.

After searching around on the web I noticed that there is information scattered about piecemeal here there, but nothing in one place, so this book is an attempt to bring together good, comprehensive and useful information on hair oils and what they can do for your hair.

Although we will be delving into the properties of many different hair oils, we also offer information on, not only *'hair oils,'* but also on *'hair'* and some of the challenges we may face in keeping it looking its best.

I hope you enjoy this 'hair oil odyssey' and that you will get some surprises and many useful pointers along the way.

*****

Contents

Chapters

1.

About Hair

2.

About Oils.

3.

Essential Oils

4.

Natural Hair Oils

Castor Oil

Coconut Oil

Evening Primrose Oil

Flaxseed Oil

Green Tea Seed Oil

Grape Seed Oil

Hemp Seed Oil

Hibiscus Flower Oil

Jojoba Oil

Kiwi Seed Oil

Kukui Seed Oil

Lavender Oil

Lemon Oil

Mango Oil

Meadowfoam Oil

Monoi Oil

Moringa Oil

Mongongo Oil

Marula Oil

Myrtle Oil

Neem Oil

Olive Oil

Pine Nut Oil

Plum Seed Oil

Peach Kernel Oil

Poppy Seed Oil

Pistachio Nut Oil

Pecan Nut Oil

Pomegranate Seed Oil

Peppermint Oil

Rosehip Oil

Rosemary Oil

Rooibos Oil

Soybean Oil

Shea Butter Oil

Sea Buckthorn Oil

Sesame Oil

Safflower Oil

Olive Squalane

Tamanu Oil

Tea Tree Oil

Ungurahua Oil

Vitamin E Oil

Wheat Germ Oil

Watermelon Seed Oil

Ximenia Oil

Ylang Ylang Oil

5.

Indian Hair Oils

Amla Oil

Brahmi Oil

Mira Oil

Trichup Oil

*****

About Hair

Why We All Need Hair Oil

Why do we all need hair oil?

Hair, like skin, needs both oil and moisture to really look and feel healthy. The lovely thing about a hair oil is that it is easily absorbed; it revives the hair while also nourishing and conditioning it!

Not only this, but there are a whole host of wonderful natural oils derived from plants and seeds or kernels and other sources that have a wide range of benefits for the health of our hair. In most cases, the oils that provide the greatest benefit are natural, organic oils.

This fact alone is an important point to keep in mind. These days our hair products are literally dripping with chemical additives and compounds that have all manner of known and unknown side effects. Many people are beginning to look for safer, simpler and more natural alternatives and hair oil, being of all-around use as a hair care product, is an obvious choice.

If you put hair oil even on your dirty hair and leave it there for several hours prior to washing it, the oil will have a deep conditioning effect and also protect the hair shafts from the stripping effects of shampoo, which in most cases are little more than glorified detergents in fancy bottles.

Not only this, but hair oil is a great 'leave-in treatment.' I have used it for the past thirty years in order to keep my course, curly mop of hair in order. Soon after I have washed my hair and it has dried naturally, I put hair oil on it and massage the oil into the scalp and then brush it through the hair. This simple technique makes it easy for me to get the brush through my tangled curls without damaging the hair. This is a personal habit, but it has worked well for me for many, many years.

Honestly, if there is one product that crosses the breadth of time, spans different continents, cultures and ethnicity's, it is the use of oil to keep the hair strong and healthy!

****

Hair Types, Which is yours?

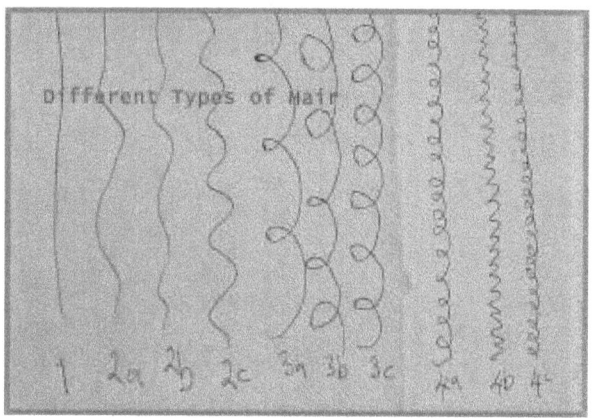

We all have somewhat distinctive hair, however, despite our unique mops, there are indicators that we can use to categorize various hair types into groups and this gives us an idea of where we are in the hair ranks among the multitudes...

We will keep things very simple here since this is not intended to be a comprehensive study on hair types, just a helpful pointer. We just need a rough outline of hair types so we can see where we best fit into the scheme of things.

Type 1. Would be the **straight** shiny hair. No curls.

Type 2. Has **moderately curly** hair in the form of a large S.

Type 3. Is **fairly dense curls** from the root to the tip.

Type 4. Is very **dense crinkled curls**. This hair type is often brittle and can break easily.

Then, of course, we have the different textures of hair.

1. The course.
2. The wiry.
3. The combination type.
4. The medium.
5. The very fine.

The variations on these themes are many.

Combination is a type that is made up of both coarse and fine hair strands and is often found in people with mixed racial backgrounds.

Wiry is most often found in African-American. The cuticles lie flat against the hair shaft giving it a glassy feel.

Course hair is the thickest of hair textures. It has a wider diameter and thicker cuticle. Because it absorbs moisture more quickly than other hair types it is also more prone to damage.

Medium textured hair is the type we find most often. In general, it is the type that also tends to wear better and withstand the rigours of day to day living.

Fine hair is more difficult to maintain and also to style and in general, requires more care and attention.

We must also take into account the amount of oil that our hair naturally contains.

Normal Hair is not greasy nor is it dry, it is the average healthy hair state, which has not been permed or coloured and generally holds its style and has a pleasant look and sheen.

Dry Hair often looks dull, it gets tangled easily, is more brittle and tends to split at the ends. Oils that stimulate the sebaceous glands in the scalp are very helpful for this hair type.

Oily Hair has the opposite problem of dry hair, these people have sebaceous glands that tend to overproduce sebum and therefore require oils that restore the glands to a more balanced level of sebum production.

So these are the basic categories of types of hair and hopefully, they will make it easier for us to slot ourselves into one of the general groups from which we can more readily move forward to discover which oil may best suit our needs and work helpfully to maximize the health of our particular hair type.

*****

Hair Health, and Beauty

Let's face it, health and beauty tend to be synonymous terms with one very much reflecting the other. Hair health and beauty are therefore very closely interlinked and looking after one tends to impact the other.

It is well known that the way our hair looks, feels and grows can change according to various environmental and health factors.

These factors include our diet, our lifestyle, the hair products we use, and even the water we shower in. If we are stressed or not getting enough sleep this will also show up in the lustre and feel of our hair.

In fact, quite aside from all the other factors that influence hair health, many of the products that we use on our hair contain the very things that cause us problems in the first place. Take Sodium Lauryl Sulfate for instance. This is one of the central ingredients of many shampoos and yet studies have shown that it actually corrodes hair follicles and impairs hair growth! Propylene Glycol is another chemical widely used in hair products and this one is known to cause rashes and skin irritations. Rather than helping us to overcome our hair problems, many of the ingredients in these products work to exacerbate them!

A little knowledge can go a long way towards helping us make the right decisions about what to use on our heads. Choosing the right oil will improve the look and feel of our hair.

We might also consider steering clear of harmful shampoos and instead use a base shampoo, to which can be added a few drops of our favourite essential oil to aid conditioning and other useful properties. This is an inexpensive and helpful move towards improving our general hair health.

It is important to have a well-rounded approach to caring for our hair. Taking note of environmental factors, the foods that we eat, what we drink and the products that we use on an almost daily basis is crucial and we need to take a good look at all of these factors.

A healthy lifestyle, adequate exercise, good dietary habits, clean water and plenty of sleep are all important factors in maintaining a healthy head of hair.

Along with careful consideration of our lifestyle habits, choosing the right oil for our hair will greatly assist us in improving and maintaining the healthful bounce of well cared for, beautiful hair.

There is no doubt about it, a lovely, healthy head of hair turns heads and this is a natural asset that we already have. It deserves our care and attention.

In the following chapters, we will examine the various Natural Oils which have been used for centuries in different countries and cultures of the world. Most of these are readily available in our local health shops and whole food stores. These oils all have specific properties and useful qualities that have proved over time to be very beneficial for the maintenance of healthy hair.

*****

About Oils

Getting into the Nitty Grities of Hair Oil

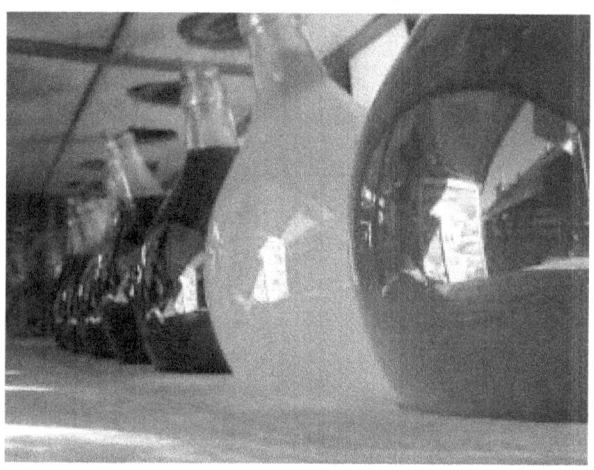

Think of all the things hair oil can do for the hair.

1. It conditions and moisturizes.

2. Adds shine and lustre.

3. Treats dandruff and numerous other annoying scalp conditions.

4. Is an excellent emollient.

5. Protects the hair from environmental extremes and harsh conditions.

6. It restores and regenerates weakened or damaged hair.

7. It nourishes the hair.

8. It takes the fizziness out of dry hair.

7. Stimulates strand growth, and the list goes on and on...

****

Basically, there are three types of oil available on the market today;

FATTY OILS, such as Castor, Shea butter etc., these are heavy oils.

SEMI FATTY OIL, such as sweet almond, avocado, sunflower etc.

These are more easily absorbed by the hair.

DRY OILS, such as grape seed, coconut, evening primrose and Jojoba oils.

These dry oils are easily absorbed by the hair and don't weigh down the hair because they are light.

What we need to determine is which hair type we have and what sort of oil is most likely to be appropriate for us in view of our hair type and lifestyle requirements. Thicker hair will generally require semi-fatty oils of the second category. Those who have very thin hair will want to use the lighter, drier hair oils.

Having determined that our hair *needs* a hair oil to maintain its health and lustre, it is a great bonus that hair oil is also effective in treating dandruff and stimulating hair growth.

Its virtues are indeed many and varied, thus, we can all benefit from adding hair oil to our list of essential grooming products because it really does deserve the title, 'Work Horse of Hair Care Products.

*****

What is the Difference between Carrier and Essential Oils?

There are basically two types of oils, Carrier, and Essential.

The Carrier Oils are normally vegetable oils which are extracted from the seeds, nuts or kernels.

1. These oils do not have a very strong potency but are mild.

2. They do not normally irritate the skin and are generally safe to use.

3. They usually have a reasonably long shelf life.

4. They do not normally evaporate when exposed to the air.

The Essential Oils, on the other hand, are usually derived from a plant's non-fatty elements such as the roots, leaves, stem, bark etc.

1. They are concentrated oils, with a high potency.

2. They should not be used directly on the skin or hair but should first be diluted before being applied.

3. They do not have a very long shelf life but degrade quickly.

4. They evaporate quickly if exposed to the air.

*****

What are Carrier Oils?

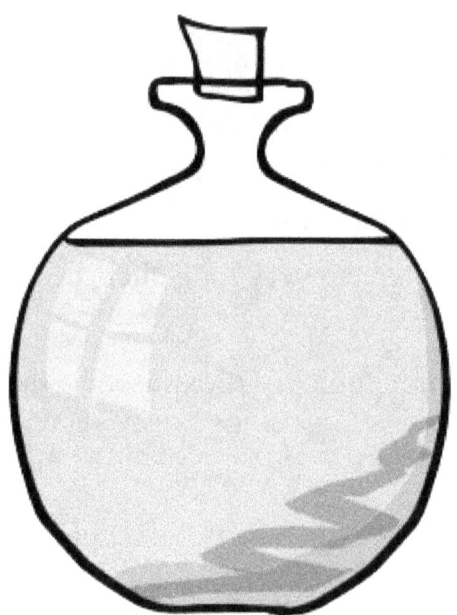

What are carrier oils and why are they important in the world of hair oils?

The so-called 'Carrier Oils' are exactly as their name suggests, they carry the oil onto the skin or hair, as the case may be. They are the oils that assist the essential oil essences in absorption. They are very important in hair care namely because they are very good moisturizers, they strengthen the hair while also nourishing the hair follicles. Where possible one should always try to use cold-pressed carrier oils.

The less processing these oils have undergone the better as this helps to retain their natural and rich nutritive value.

As well as their high absorption properties, many of the carrier oils are also known to have anti-bacterial and anti-fungal properties and are said to have a chemical signalling effect that enhances metabolism.

Examples of Carrier Oils.

Sunflower Oil has high levels of oleic acid and is known to be deeply nourishing.

Olive Oil: the cold-pressed version is good and the greener it is in colour, the better. This oil has many beneficial properties useful in general hair care.

Coconut Oil is a mild and all-around hair oil.

Castor Oil acts as a protective medium against harsh environmental conditions and has many other benefits besides.

Avocado Oil is a nutrient-rich and organic oil with great nourishing effects on the hair.

Jojoba Oil is famous for its lightness it's high absorption properties and nutrient-rich profile.

Sweet Almond Oil: soften, soothes and conditions.

Vitamin E Oil is a highly nourishing and nutrient-rich oil.

Apricot Oil: a great all-round carrier oil and particularly useful for ageing and more mature skin and scalp types.

Argan Oil is rich in anti-oxidants and is known to have wonderful absorption properties.

Wheat Germ Oil: Unrefined and cold-pressed this oil has numerous beneficial effects in hair and skin care.

Other carrier oils include the following;

Soybean Oil:

Cherry Seed Oil:

Shea Butter Oil

Peach Kernel Oil:

Poppy Seed Oil:

Grape Seed Oil:

Safflower Oil:

Olive Squalene:

This is by no means an exhaustive list of **carrier oils**, but these are the ones most widely known and available. A more comprehensive examination of their properties and usefulness in hair care is set out for readers in the Natural Hair Oils section below.

*****

Essential Oils

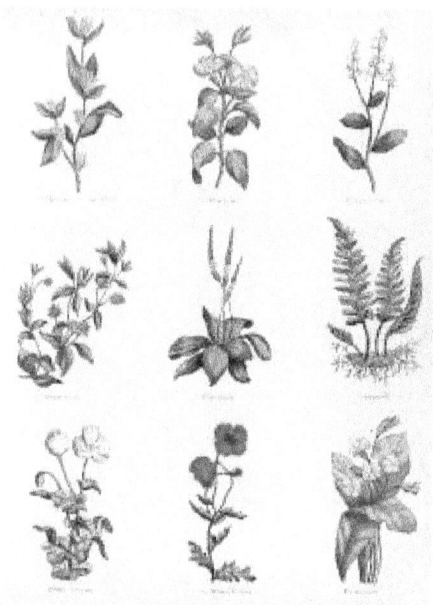

An Overview of Essential oils.

It is not always necessary to buy the most expensive oil on the market to get the best product for our hair! Essential oils are very concentrated distillations of plants and herbs such as Lavender, Rosemary, Peppermint, and Carrot, to name a few.

These natural oils, which are easily and affordably available to us at our local health food shop or whole food retailer, offer some remarkable properties and have proved, over the course of time, just how useful and effective they can be.

According to our hair type and individual needs, the essential oils most useful for the hair are as follows;

Normal hair can benefit from;

Lavender

Rosemary

Thyme

Cedarwood

Lemon

Geranium

Chamomile

Clary Sage

Dry hair will find the following oils beneficial;

Rosemary

Lavender

Geranium

Sandalwood

Myrrh

Peppermint

Oily Hair responds well to the following oils;

Rosemary

Lavender
Peppermint
Tea Tree
Patchouli
Lemongrass
Ylang Ylang

As you can see the list is extensive and I am sure there are many more essential oils out there that are useful in maintaining good hair health but this should give the reader an idea of the oils most commonly used and for which hair types.

Just ahead we will discuss the types of hair problems and conditions for which various essential oils have been found to be effective so that you can further assess which ones might be useful to you.

*****

What the Essential Oils Can Do For Your Hair.

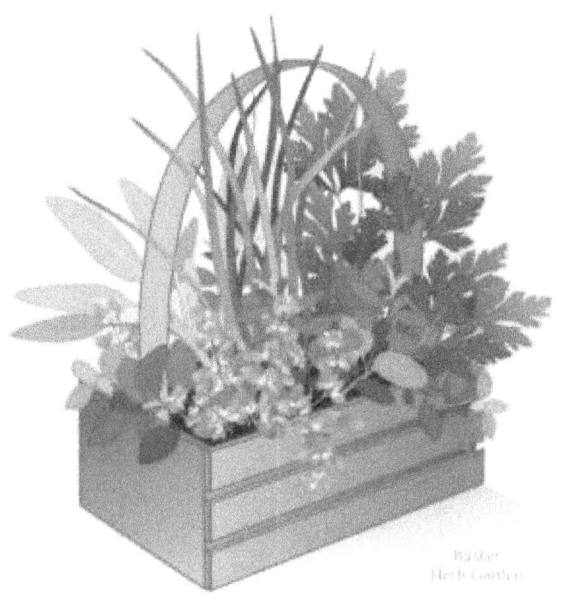

Essential Oils have a long history of usefulness in the hair care domain.

A few drops of one of these concentrated oil essences will greatly enhance the effectiveness of a base shampoo or carrier oil.

A carrier oil, by the way, is an oil that can act as a base for essential oils, or also be used as a stand-alone oil on the hair. It has high absorption properties and assists in the assimilation of essential oils.

The essential oils are the concentrated active ingredients in natural hair oil combinations and because they are so concentrated, it is important to remember that one can overdo their use. Just a few drops, added to a base oil will greatly enhance its effectiveness.

Here are a few of the common problems associated with Hair and Scalp care and the essential oils that have proved to be most useful in eliminating them.

Hair Loss and Hair Thinning

Cedarwood has anti-bacterial properties and is useful in eliminating scalp infections that might be inhibiting normal hair growth.

Carrot Root, this oil detoxifies and stimulates skin and hair follicle regrowth.

Cypress increases circulation and capillary strength.

Rosemary is well known for its hair growth-enhancing properties.

Sage also has well known stimulating properties that promote hair growth.

Basil promotes hair growth.

Thyme is also known to be beneficial in treating hair loss.

Clove may well be one of the most effective oils in the treatment of hair loss.

Chamomile.

Dry Hair.

Myrrh is effective for dry hair.

Peppermint.

Lavender.

Rosemary.

Cedarwood.

Dandruff.

Lavender is a good all-rounder. It has anti-inflammatory and anti-bacterial properties useful in the treatment of dandruff.

Sage balances scalp oils and is useful in normalizing sebum production.

Tea Tree, effective in the treatment of dry scalp, dandruff, and lice.

Myrrh treats dandruff.

Rosemary is also effective.

Ylang Ylang, another all-rounder, is also useful in the treatment of dandruff.

Eucalyptus, with its antiseptic properties, is useful as a dandruff treatment.

Greasy Hair.

Basil has slightly astringent properties.

Cedarwood helps to balance the scalp oils.

Lemon apart from giving pleasing highlights to the hair, lemon is also astringent and has balancing properties for the scalp oils.

Lemon Grass

Patchouli

Ylang Ylang

Myrtle helps to balance scalp oils.

Split Ends.

Rosemary

Burdock, a great oil in helping to control hair breakage.

Lavender

Chamomile

Peppermint

Frizzy Hair.

Bay Leaf energizes and helps to thin hair.

Chamomile has calming and balancing properties.

Clary Sage is a truly all-round essential hair oil.

Carrot Root

Geranium, apart from having a very pleasant scent, this oil balances, and calms.

Juniper Berry has cleansing and calming qualities.

Lemon Verbena is a great hair tonic.

As you can see, the essential, natural oils can play a very important role in good hair health and care and as we mentioned earlier they are affordable and easily available. They are definitely worth experimenting with for those who are interested in putting together their own home formulations.

*****

The Essential Oils That Increase Hair Growth

When it comes to hair oils, as we have seen earlier, we can break them down into two basic categories.

The **carrier oils**, which are a type of base oil that quite literally carry their own and the essential oils, nutritive values into the hair shaft and skin.

The **essential oils**, which are volatile, concentrated natural oils. The carrier oils are normally mild and can be used directly on the skin, hair and scalp, but the essential oils should always be diluted and just a few drops will normally suffice.

We have given a comprehensive list of both carrier and essential oils, describing the oils that have been found to be most beneficial in hair and skin care. They all differ in their potency of essential fatty acids, compounds and anti-oxidants and this is what gives them their own unique properties and usefulness.

When it comes to increasing the hair growth one needs to find an oil that contains at least one, if not all of the following properties. However, as many of the oils contain some, but not all of the following properties, one can mix a carrier oil, for example, coconut, olive or safflower oil, with a few drops of one or two essential oils to get the desired potency and combination.

A hair oil combination that will optimize hair growth or regrowth should include all of the following properties.

The most useful oils to increase hair growth;

1. Should stimulate blood circulation to the scalp.

2. Should be an oil that contains high nutritive values.

3. Should have properties that help to balance the natural oils on the scalp.

4. Should support and boost the Immune System.

Stimulating Essential Oils

The stimulating essential oils are the ones that increase the metabolic rate at the cellular level thereby promoting hair growth. They also normally contain organic signalers called key-tones. These work to ratchet up the cellular metabolic process and enhance hair growth and hair health.

Some of the oils which contain these properties are Rosemary, Cloves, Clary Sage and Cedarwood.

Balancing Essential Oils

These are essential oils that facilitate the balancing and normalization of sebum production on the scalp. These oils have a soothing and balancing action the hormones. They reduce inflammation, soothe the hair follicle and decrease irritation on the scalp, thereby paving the way for a healthy hair growing environment.

Some of the essential oils that contain these properties are Lavender, Lemon oil and Green Myrtle.

Nutritive Oils

These oils provide;

1. Necessary essential fatty acids which make it possible for the oil to be absorbed and assimilated into the hair shaft.

2. Anti-oxidants in the form of vitamins and minerals, all of which neutralize the oxidation process which gradually depletes the mitochondria within the hair follicle, thereby weakening it. Oxidation is an ongoing process that is greatly accelerated by some factors. These include the types of foods we eat, our lifestyle habits, sleep, exercise, and the chemicals in personal care products that we use on a daily basis and so on.

Some of the oils that contain these properties are Cloves, which incidentally contains the highest known anti-oxidant profile of any other plant-based oil, Carrot Root, Cedarwood.

Many carrier oils also contain highly nutritive properties. Some examples are Jojoba, Coconut oil, Red Palm Oil, Olive oil, Safflower oil, to name just a few.

Immune Supportive or Booster Oils

These oils primarily treat scalp and skin infections which greatly hinder hair growth. Such essential oils have a number of important properties such as being, anti-inflammatory, anti-bacterial, and anti-fungal and so on. Some of the oils that contain these properties are Green Myrtle, Cedarwood and Cloves and Lemon oil.

All of these oils are discussed in greater detail individually in the categories dealing with **essential oils** and **natural hair oils** further on.

These days many, many products are available on the market and a lot of them contain chemical compounds that may well exacerbate hair and scalp problems. This is why a little knowledge gives us great power and these days we have it all at our fingertips. Not only can we save a considerable amount of money, but we do ourselves a great favour by limiting the levels of toxins to which we expose ourselves.

The essential and natural hair oils are all plant-based, natural oils. When purchasing and where ever possible one should choose, cold-pressed and organic brands that have the greatest chance of retaining their optimum nutritive and healing values.

Good health and happy hair growing!

*****

Natural Hair Oils

In the following section, we will examine the oils that have proven to be most effective when it comes to Hair Health and Maintenance.

Argan Oil, Liquid Gold

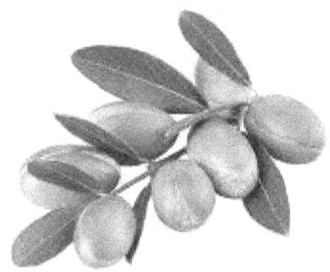

Argan oil is the recent 'darling' and discovery of the western world.

The Argan tree grows in South-Western Morocco, a rare and precious tree that takes many, many years to grow and produce its fruit. In former times, it was known to grow over a wide area of Northern Africa, but now it can only be found in the south-western regions. For this reason, there is a strong and growing movement to help conserve not only the trees but also the eco-system in which they grow.

Touted as one of nature's richest moisturizers, Argan Oil is not only packed with fatty acids but is so lightweight that it does not leave a greasy film on the skin or hair and is easily absorbed by skin and hair follicles. In fact, it absorbs almost instantly, deeply conditioning the hair and adding extra elasticity to damaged and dry hair.

Berber women have traditionally harvested and used Argan Oil for many centuries. The old system of harvesting the Argan nuts was a very long and labor-intensive process. In most areas, however, this has now changed and the nuts, which are hand-picked from the trees and not the ground, are carefully put through a more modern hand and machine cold-pressing process that extracts the extra-virgin Argan Oil with the least damage to its natural state.

If one intends to try this oil, prior to buying one should always check the list of ingredients on the bottle's label before deciding to make any purchase.

There are also a few other things to keep in mind. 100% pure is best, avoid anything with 'added Argan oil' written on the label.

When checking out different Argan oil products always look at the colour and go for oils that have a rich golden hue.

It should also have a light nutty odour to it. Argan is a vegetable oil and that nutty aroma is a sign of authenticity. Over-processing will tend to change the colour and smell of this oil from its natural state so avoid anything that is without its natural scent or which is dull coloured. We want an oil that is rich and has a creamy consistency.

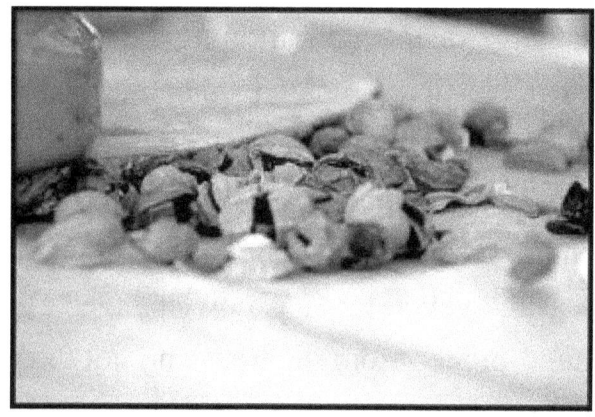

Photo Credit: Avi Paz. www.flickr.com/photos/pazavi. Creative Commons

Argan oil is one of the rarest and most precious oils available on the market today and as such it does not come cheap. So take special care to make sure that you get the best and most authentic product possible.

Sweet Almond Oil, a Treat for your Hair

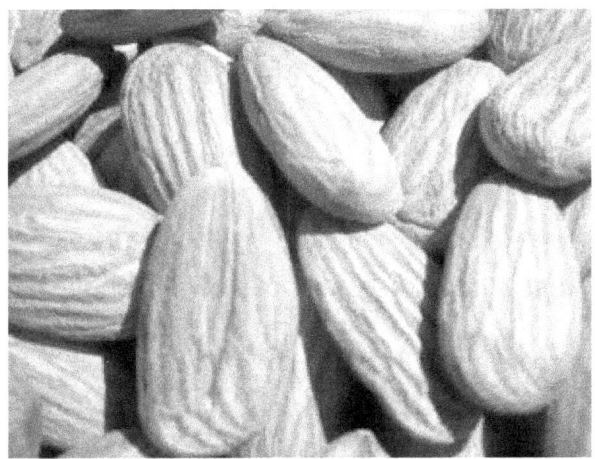

Photo Credit: Health Aliciousness. www.flickr.com/photos/healthaliciousness. Creative Commons

Sweet Almond Oil is a treat for your hair, quite literally. This is another excellent 'carrier oil'. It is nutrient-rich and a good moisturizing oil that absorbs easily and gives many benefits to both hair and skin.

If a few drops of an appropriate essential oil such as Rosemary, are added to Sweet Almond and then massaged thoroughly into the scalp it will greatly assist in stimulating the circulation of blood over the scalp, enhancing the health of both scalp and hair and thereby assisting in promoting hair growth.

It is widely available, but always try to buy an organic, cold-pressed and certified brand. Check the label carefully and be sure to note the expiry date.

Almond oil does not have a very long shelf life so anything that is over a year old should most certainly be avoided.

If you buy organic Sweet Almond oil it will have a slightly thick consistency and this is something to look out for when purchasing this product and will be an indicator of quality.

Sweet Almond oil is a nut-based oil and therefore should be used with caution by those who have known allergies.

*****

Apricot Kernel Oil

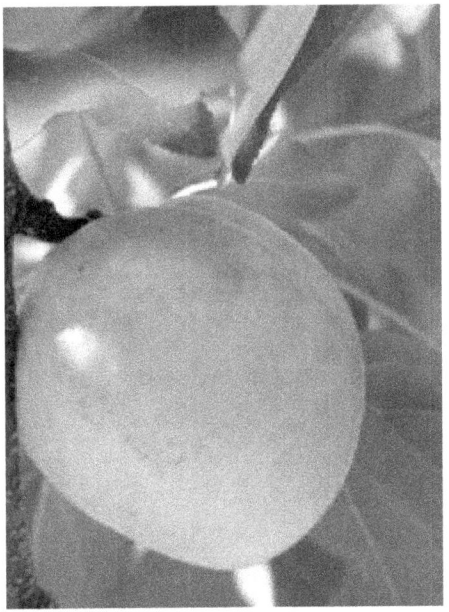

Photo Credit: Lepre Chaun HR. www.flickr.com/photos/leprechaunhr. Creative Commons

Apricot Kernel Oil is somewhat similar to Sweet Almond and Peach oil in both appearance and viscosity. It is extracted from the kernel of the apricot fruit and is a highly nutritive oil. Apricot oil is also noted to be of particular use as a healing oil when massaged into the scalp.

Properties. It is low in saturated fat but contains more than 65% essential fatty acids which are particularly beneficial in skin and hair care. Contains numerous anti-oxidants, particularly Vitamin E.

Benefits for Hair

1. Absorbs easily without leaving any greasy residue on the skin or hair.
2. An effective conditioner and moisturizer for hair.
3. It is an emollient.
4. Helps to restore and protect damaged or weakened hair.
5. Helps to limit the damage of split ends.
6. Adds shine and lustre to the hair.
7. Highly nutritive leave-in oil for hair.
8. Anti-fungal and anti-inflammatory properties make this an effective oil in treating scalp conditions such as dandruff and psoriasis.

Shelf Life. Apricot Kernel oil has an approximate shelf life of twelve months.

Side Effects. Anyone with known allergies to nuts should exercise caution where the use of nut-based oils is concerned, however, Apricot oil is thought to be a milder alternative for people who experience allergies along with the use of such oils as Sweet Almond oil.

*****

Avocado Oil

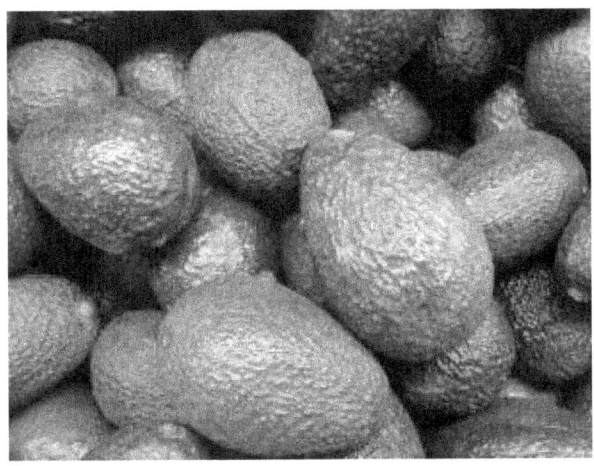

Photo Credit. Olle Svensson.www.flickr.com/photos/ollesvensson. Creative Commons

Avocado oil is a great 'all-round', nutrient-rich hair oil of a slightly heavy consistency, more suitable for people with thicker hair types. This oil is a very good moisturizer and will absorb easily and quickly into the hair and the skin without leaving a greasy film on the surface.

This is one of our great 'super foods'. Avocados are packed with nutrients, both minerals and vitamins. Because of these properties, it is important to always look for a good cold-pressed brand if you are going to purchase this oil. The cold-pressing process will help to retain the natural nutrients in the oil which heating would otherwise destroy.

The great thing about Avocado oil is its very high content of mono-unsaturated fatty acids. This is the unique and most potent aspect of Avocado oil. When it comes to hair care, mono-unsaturated fatty acids in an oil, are of great benefit. These fatty acids condition, they protect, they nourish and they also help to unclog hair follicles and thereby balance the scalp's natural oils and promote healthy hair growth.

There can be no doubt about it, Avocado oil is a very valuable carrier oil for the hair. It is not as costly as other, and perhaps now more famous types of oils, but it is every bit as beneficial and with regular use, you will soon come to understand why it is a great oil and one to consider using regularly.

*****

Babassu Oil

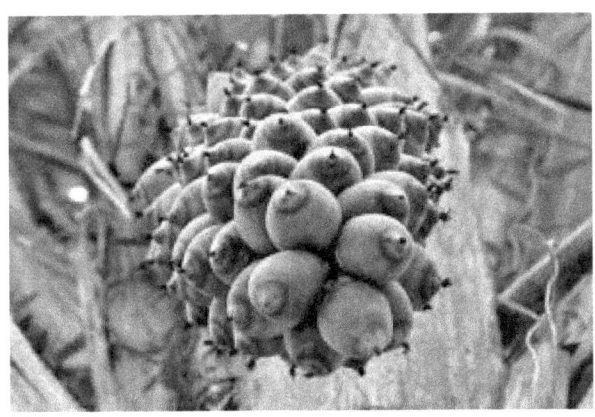

Photo Credit. Confessions of a Blog Vixen.
www.confessionsofablogvixen.com. Creative Commons.
Babassu Oil which is also known by the name of Cusi Oil
is a vegetable oil that is extracted from the seeds of the
Babassu Palm which grow in the forests of the Amazon.
This oil is used in cooking but has recently also become
known as a valuable and useful oil for cosmetic preparations
that can be used on hair and skin. There are many
similarities between Babbasu oil and Coconut oil.

Properties. Babassu oil contains an approximate 70%
lipid profile. It has numerous essential fatty acids including
lauric acid, myristic acid and oleic acids to name a few.

Benefits for Hair.

1. Acts as an emollient.

2. Rehydrates the hair and is an effective conditioner and moisturizer.

3. Nourishes the skin and hair follicles with its numerous nutrients.

4. Is known for its regenerating properties.

5. Balances the sebum secretion and scalp oil production.

6. Leaves no greasy residue and is completely absorbed.

7. Has exfoliating properties that assist in the removal of residues and build-up on the hair and skin leaving it soft and shiny.

Shelf Life. This is a stable oil and has an approximate shelf life of between one and two years if stored properly.

Indications. There are no known side effects associated with the use of this oil but as we always advise, care should be taken when known allergies are present.

*****

Baobab Oil

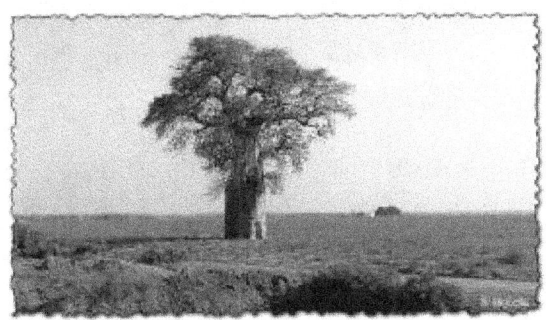

Photo Credit. Ismail Mia. www.flickr.com/photos/bigdmia. Creative Commons

Baobab Oil is extracted from the fruit of the Baobab Tree which grows in southern and eastern Africa. It is known primarily for its impressive moisturizing properties and used widely on hair and skin. However, it is also known to have many other healing qualities associated with skin and hair conditions, such as acne, scars, eczema, psoriasis and the list goes on.

This oil is known to absorb quickly into the skin and hair shafts and makes a great natural moisturizer but it does far more than this. It really is an oil with amazing properties.

Interestingly the essential fatty acids of this oil are found to be almost double those present in the now famous 'Argan

Oil'. That is, its Omega and Palmitic oil content, not to mention the well known nutritive values of Baobab Oil.

Baobab oil is derived from the seeds of the Baobab fruit and is a rich and golden coloured oil. It absorbs quickly and easily without clogging the pores or leaving behind traces of greasiness. It is packed with anti-oxidants and known for its remarkable anti-ageing and regenerating properties.

The oil is cold-pressed from the seeds and has a long shelf life of two years. It is a somewhat costly oil but given its concentrated composition, one can use it sparingly and also add a few drops of it to enrich other carrier oils thus making the oil last much longer.

This is definitely an oil to look out for.

*****

Black Seed Oil

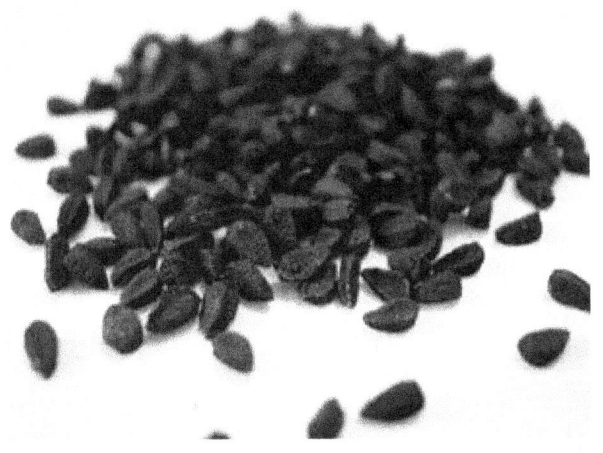

Black Seed Oil is derived from the seeds of the Black Seed plant and has a deep gold, sometimes a darkish brown, or even black appearance as an oil.

It has a long and much-respected history in medicinal circles and was used even back in Egyptian times where it was discovered in a number of famous Pharaoh's tombs.

Properties. The oil from Black Seed, otherwise known as Nigella Sativa, is a great conditioner and moisturizer for hair and skin and is a very concentrated source of essential fatty acids.

Black Seed oil packs 85% anti-oxidant load and above 30% in essential fatty acids.

Benefits for Hair.

1. This oil can be used to help heal dry scalp, psoriasis, and other such scalp conditions.

2. It has also been shown to be beneficial for people who are recovering from hair loss after cancer treatments.

3. This is a completely natural oil with no chemical additives and its regular use on the hair, skin and scalp is a great support to an impaired immune system, assisting in a speedy recovery and the quick regrowth of hair.

4. An effective conditioner and moisturizer for skin and hair.

Shelf Life. When properly stored one can expect this oil to have a shelf life of approximately two years.

Side Effects. Used as an external oil there are no known indications associated with its use, but where there are known allergies one should, as always, exercise caution.

*****

Brazil Nut Oil

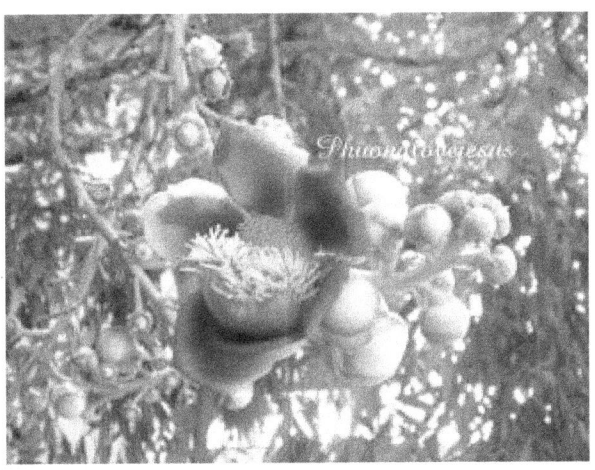

Photo Credit. Vietnam Plants and the USA Plants. www.flickr.com/photos/zoyachubby. Creative Commons

Brazil Nut Oil derives from the Brazilian Nut Tree, a native of South America. Although the tree grows widely both in its pristine forests and suburban and rural areas, it is only from the trees in the forest that the flowers of the trees are pollinated and thus produce the fruit which in turn produce the nuts.

Because the whole chain of interdependencies for producing the nuts and in turn the oil is a very delicate one, widespread production of the Brazil Nut can be variable and often not reliable. It grows only in South America and if a season fails, availability can be scarce.

Properties. The oil is nutrient-rich, particularly in the Omega 6 fatty acids. It has a rich and creamy feel due to its high-fat content and makes for a very luxurious oil with great moisturizing properties. It also contains notably high quantities of selenium.

It has certainly become a favourite for various cosmetic uses.

Benefits for Hair.

1. In the realm of hair care, Brazil Nut oil has shown itself to be useful in the treatment of dandruff and psoriasis.

2. If regularly massaged into the scalp it assists in the natural production of sebum and balances the oils at the hair roots, creating a healthy environment for hair growth and hair health.

3. It has regenerative qualities that strengthen and protect weakened and damaged hair.

4. It adds lustre and enhances the hair's natural colour.

5. It is a very rich oil and its high nutritive content make it an especially effective conditioner that not only moisturizes but also nourishes the hair.

6. This is also an effective emollient oil that coats and protects the hair from harsh environmental factors, such as

heat, cold, wind and dry conditions. It also adds protection from pollutants.

Shelf Life. This is a relatively stable oil but due to its high percentage of polyunsaturated fatty acids, once a bottle is opened it is advised to store this oil in the fridge to maximize its shelf life. When stored properly it should have a shelf life of at least one year.

Side Effects. Those with known allergic sensitivities should avoid using this Brazil Nut oil until you have tested yourself for possible reactions. It has been noted that these nuts contain an amount of radium.

*****

Broccoli Seed Oil

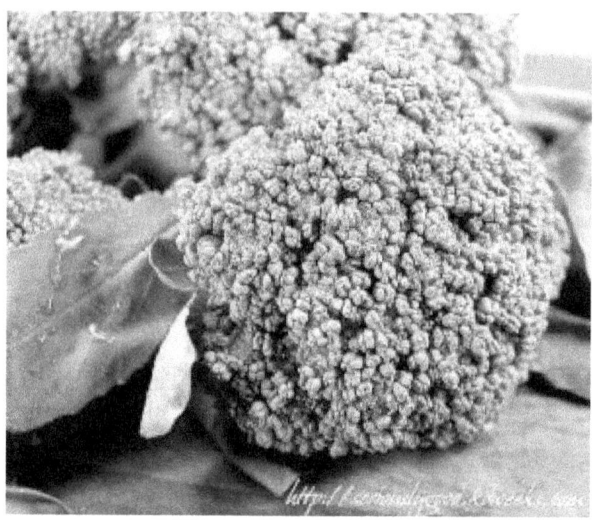

Photo Credit. Seriously Good 1. www.flickr.com/photos/68188294@N00. Creative Commons

Broccoli Seed Oil is becoming known as a natural alternative to the use of silicon in shampoos, conditioners and hair styling gels. This oil adds a sheen and lustre to the hair that is normally achieved by the use of chemical additives in hair care products.

Properties. This oil has a unique fatty acid composition. It contains Omega 9 fatty acids which are the component that imparts a 'shine' to the hair. It also contains many other essential fatty acids and anti-oxidants. The Vitamin most prevalent in this oil is Vitamin A, (Retinol). It has approximately an 85% per cent load of Polyunsaturated fatty acids.

Benefits for Hair.

1. This is an effective hydrating oil.

2. It is non-greasy and absorbs easily and quickly without leaving any film or trace on the hair or skin.

3. Highly nourishing oil.

4. A great moisturizer and conditioner.

5. Adds a sheen and lustre to the hair which is comparable to that produced by silicon but without the chemical side effects.

6. Protects all types of hair from environmental factors that could dry or strip the hair.

7. Assists in the hairs regeneration and overall health.

Shelf Life. Broccoli Seed oil has a shelf life of approximately one year.

Side Effects. There are no noted indications associated with the use of this oil. However as is always advised, where known allergies are present, exercise caution.

*****

Camellia Seed Oil

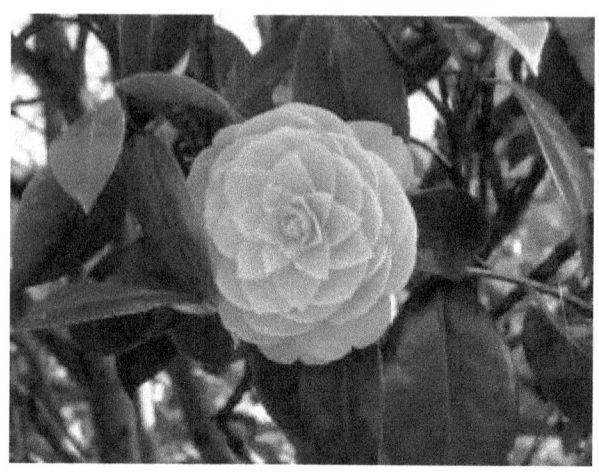

Photo Credit. V.A. Yardley.www.flickr.com/photos/vayardley. Creative Commons

Camellia Seed Oil is an exotic and rich oil that absorbs into the skin and hair quickly without leaving greasy traces.

It has an eighty plus per cent composition of fatty acids, namely mono-unsaturated oleic acid, making it a nutrition-packed oil with wonderful conditioning and moisturizing properties.

This oil has a faint herbal aroma and has a clear golden hue. It has a long shelf life which makes it a great product for hair and skin care creams and potions.

Camellia seed oil has long been used as a culinary oil in the South of China and is known to have a number of beneficial health effects. It should also be mentioned that Camellia Oil is often confused with Tea Seed oil, but they are both from different families of Camellia. Camellia oil is from the olifera family while tea seed oil is derived from Camellia sinensis.

The list of benefits one can derive from using this oil as a skin and hair care product is long and well worth taking note of. Here are just a few;

Benefits for Hair.

1. It is said to promote hair growth.

2. Heals various scalp conditions.

3. It is a great conditioner as we already noted.

4. Also acts as an emollient blocking out pollutants and harmful UV rays.

This is an all-round product for skin and hair care.

****

Carrot Oil

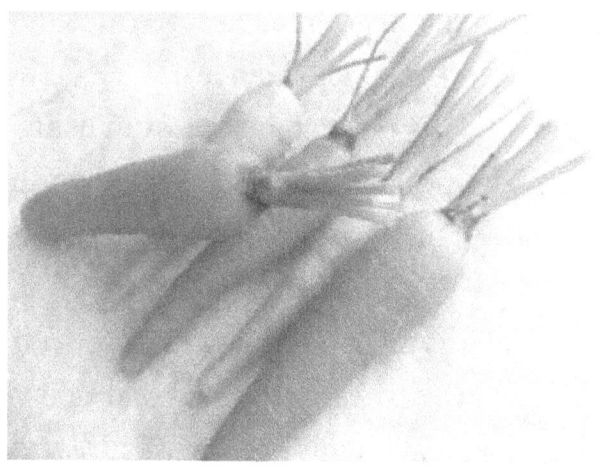

Photo Credit. Chris Cook. www.flickr.com/photos/clcphoto. Creative Commons

Carrot Oil is a highly nourishing essential oil with lots of anti-oxidants, most notably Beta- Carotene of Vitamin A fame. This oil is derived from Daucus Carota, a form of wild carrot. There are two kinds of carrot oil, one is extracted from the seeds, the other from the roots. Both are nutrient heavy oils with many benefits for both hair and skin.

Properties. Very high in carotene's which are the precursors of vitamin A. The oil also has a high Vitamin E content and other minerals and nutrients that are beneficial for both skin and hair.

Benefits for Hair.

1. Foremost among other essential oils in skin cell regeneration; it can be massaged into the scalp after it has been diluted with a carrier oil of your choice.

2. Moisturizes and Conditions the hair.

3. Nourishes the hair shaft and strengthens it.

4. Assists in enhancing the highlights of one's natural hair colour.

5. This oil helps to balance the scalp oils.

6. Effective in the treatment of psoriasis, dandruff, and scalp irritations.

Side Effects. Carrot oil is generally regarded as a safe oil, but it should be avoided during pregnancy and where known allergies are present.

*****

Cedarwood Oil

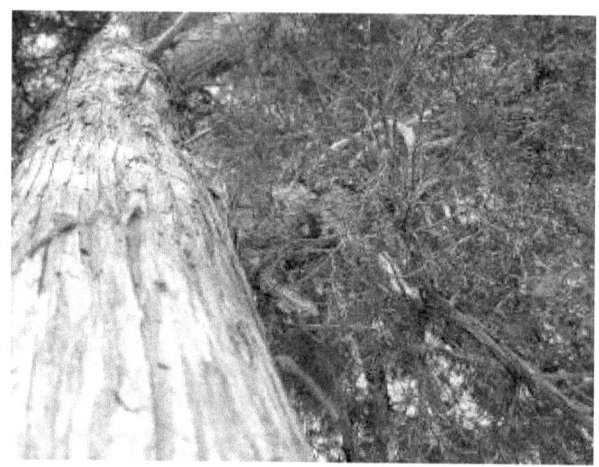

Photo Credit. Trek kyandy. www.flickr.com/photos/trekkyandy.Creative Commons.

Cedar Wood Oil is another of the essential oils that is beneficial for treating several hair care conditions. The oil has a clean and fresh fragrance and is derived from the foliage and on occasion the wood and roots of various kinds of Conifer Trees.

Properties. Among several properties, it is known to be anti-fungal, anti-bacterial, anti-septic and there is also mention of its being an effective insecticide. This oil also contains astringent properties.

Benefits for Hair.

1. Soothes irritations and itching of the scalp.

2. Effective in the treatment of scalp conditions such as dandruff.

3. When massaged into the scalp, not only relieves the discomfort of scalp oil imbalances but calms and eases the scalp and nerve endings.

4. Is known to be effective in the treatment of psoriasis.

5. Helpful in controlling and removing infestations of head lice and nits.

6. Excellent at stimulating and oxygenating the hair roots and follicles, thus promoting hair growth and general scalp health.

7. Useful in the treatment and prevention of hair loss.

8. Adds lustre and shine to the hair.

Side Effects. It is advised that children and pregnant women should avoid the use of Cedarwood oil. It should always be diluted before applying externally in order to avoid irritation and skin reactions.

*****

Cherry Seed Oil

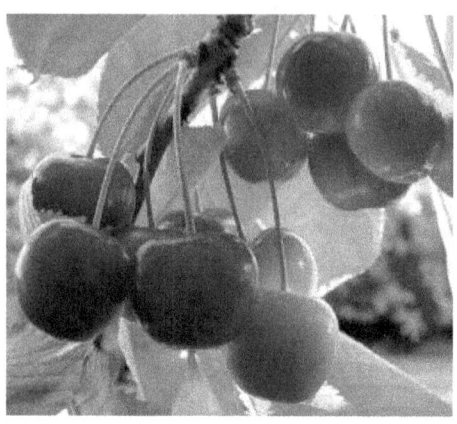

Photo Credit. D.H.Wright. www.flickr.com/photos/dhwright. Creative Commons

Cherry Seed Oil is a nutrient-rich hair oil that can be used as a carrier or base oil to which essential oils may be added or it can be simply used by itself.

Properties. This oil is high in polyunsaturated fatty acids. It contains many essential fatty acids, particularly oleic acid, and eleostearic acid. It also contains antioxidants such as Vitamins A and E but is particularly noted for its high natural Vitamin A content.

There are quite a few similarities between Cherry Seed oil and the properties contained in Sweet Almond Oil although

Cherry Kernel is lighter and more easily absorbed by skin and hair.

Benefits for Hair.

1. The oil is a rich emollient and its high levels of oleic acid greatly assist in the assimilation and absorption of the oil and nutrients directly into the cells.

2. It is a very effective conditioner.

3. Highly nutritious oil for skin and hair.

4. Is known to contain properties that protect against harmful UV rays and environmental pollutants.

5. Is useful in the treatment of scalp and skin conditions. Its anti-inflammatory properties reduce inflammation and irritation to the skin and scalp

6. Rehydrates the hair and skin and protects it from further drying effects of wind, sun, and cold.

Other Uses. It is also an oil that has a pleasant fragrance and for this reason, is often used as a carrier oil in aromatherapy and for massage treatments.

Shelf Life. This is a stable oil with an approximate 12-month shelf life.

*****

Clary Sage Oil

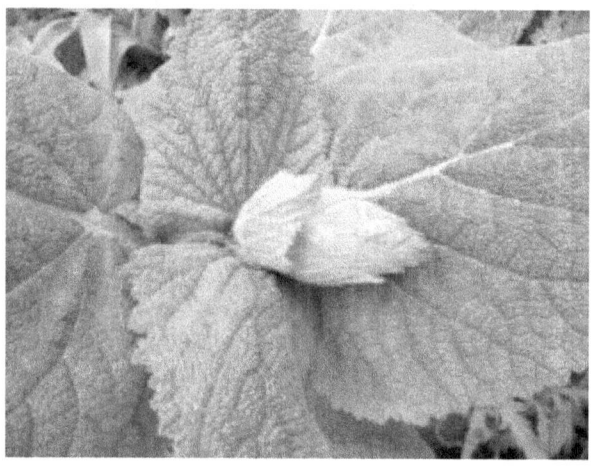

Photo Credit. Wally Grom.www.flickr.com/photos/33037982@N04/. Creative Commons

Clary Sage Oil has rejuvenating properties and is also used to assist in balancing hormones.

Properties. This essential oil is high in anti-oxidants.

Benefits for Hair.

1. This oil is said to boost hair growth.

2. Strengthen the hair from the cellular level.

3. Prevents premature hair loss.

4. Helps to balance the scalp oils.

5. Stimulates the scalp and hair follicles, increasing blood circulation and enhancing normal hair growth.

6. Helps to make the hair manageable and adds lustre and shine.

7. Helps to prevent dandruff.

8. Clary Sage oil is an overall great hair tonic.

Side Effects. No known toxicity but should be avoided during pregnancy.

*****

Cloves

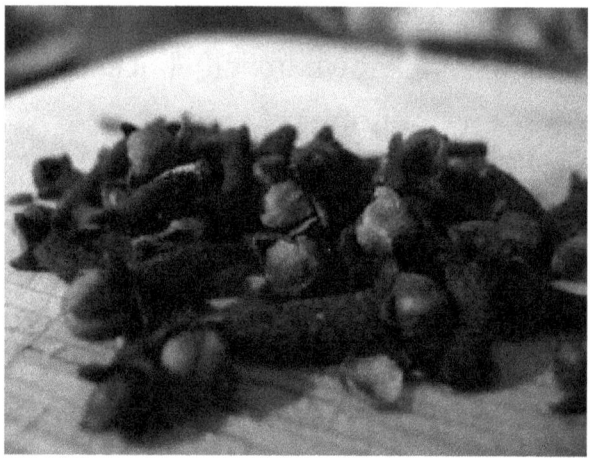

Photo Credit. Elana Dan. www.flickr.com/photos/melintur. Creative Commons

Clove Oil is one of the essential oils that appears to have endless applications and uses. It is also a very important oil for the hair.

Benefits for Hair. As many skin and hair conditions are due to poor diet and the use of chemical compounds in our day-to-day personal care products, it is always important to address the underlying conditions that are exacerbating a scalp or hair problem. However, Clove oil, which is a powerful anti-fungal and anti-bacterial oil is an excellent natural treatment.

1. The oil is packed with anti-oxidants which are very nourishing for the hair.
2. Stimulates the blood circulation in and around the hair follicles enhancing hair growth.
3. Effectively treats scalp conditions such as dandruff, dry flaky scalp and so on.

Side Effects. This is a very potent oil and one should exercise care with its use. Children should not take it internally and pregnant women advised to avoid its use during their term.

******

Cranberry Seed Oil

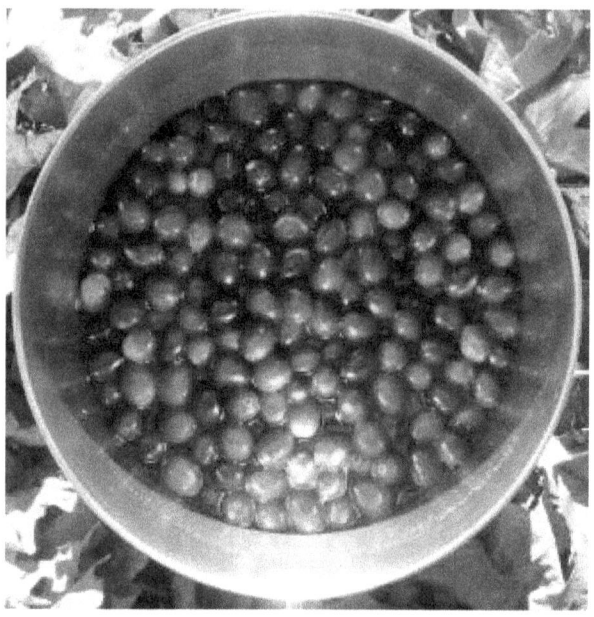

Cranberry Seed Oil is quickly acquiring a reputation as an oil that bestows many benefits for the hair and the skin. It has some unique properties that make it a valuable addition to skin and hair care products. The seeds of the cranberry used to be thrown away but now it is known just how nutrient-rich they are and how many health benefits the oil from these seeds can bestow, they are very much utilized and provide an important contribution to skin and hair care products.

Properties. This is a nutrient-rich oil that contains a significant number of Anti-oxidants such as Vitamins E and A. In fact of all the vegetable oils, Cranberry seed oil contains the highest proportion of tocotrienols and tocopherols which are found the Vitamin E. It is also said to contain many essential fatty acids and particularly the EFAs, Omega3, 6 and 9, which are not normally present in other oils.

Benefits for Hair.

1. This oil is an excellent moisturizer that absorbs quickly and carries its nutrient load swiftly into the hair shaft.

2. It has also shown itself to be very helpful in the treatment of scalp conditions such as Psoriasis, dandruff, and scaly scalp. So, one can count on the benefits of healing, strengthening and moisturizing with this oil.

3. High Anti-oxidant content, particularly Vitamins A and E.

4. Unusually high in Essential Fatty Acids. As these EFAs are not normally produced by our bodies and yet essential in maintaining the health and elasticity of our skin and hair, this oil provides a valuable source of these nutrients.

5. Re-hydrates the hair shaft and protects it from damaging environmental conditions.

Other Uses. The oil is also widely appreciated in skin care products for its moisturizing properties and is also said to be an excellent skin prophylactic in that it can delay and even prevent irritating skin condition from developing.

Shelf Life. Due to its high Anti-Oxidant content, this oil is stable and has a long shelf life of approximately two years. Because of this property, it is also used to help 'carry' less stable oils.

Indications. No known indications but as with the use of all oils, if you have known allergies then caution should be exercised when using the oil.

*****

Castor Oil, the Great All-Rounder

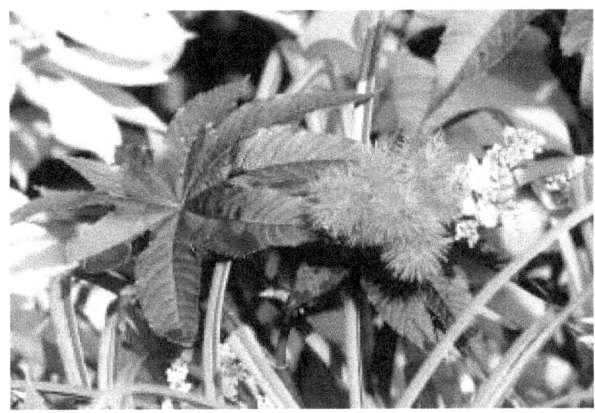

Photo Credit. Piers Nye. www.flickr.com/photos/piers_nye. Creative Commons

Castor oil is a great all-rounder for hair, although one might be forgiven for never having considered it in that light.

This oil was something that was always sitting in a corner of our bathroom cupboard when I was growing up. If we had stomach problems or something along those lines, the Castor oil came out of its hiding place and we had to gulp down a few spoonful's of it. This is not an easy oil to get down...

With this sort of association attached to it while I was growing up, it was not one of my favourite oils.

I would never have thought of it as a valuable carrier oil for hair! But there it is. Good old, boring Castor oil is a truly amazing substance with many different uses and applications.

Benefits for Hair

1. For the hair, it is a valuable emollient and helps it to retain its natural moisture.

2. It also has anti-fungal, anti-viral and anti-bacterial properties. And, and, and... The list goes on. The oil is multifunctional and is very much worthy of recognition as a valuable carrier oil for hair.

Castor oil is derived from the seeds of the Castor plant, and various grades of this oil are used in anything from motor lubrication through to numerous medicinal uses.

With regards to hair care, it has been noted, that where there is hair loss or thinning, this oil is said to have a beneficial effect. In cases where there are itchiness and dryness of the scalp, it shines, yet again, as an effective treatment and it is known to have a natural anti-microbial effect.

Now it's not the sexiest oil in the world to use... It is thick and it can feel sticky and not very pleasant to the touch.

However, there are a few tricks that will make the experience of giving your hair a good old Castor oil treatment, somewhat more comfortable. We will mention a few of those later.

Castor oil is not a moisturizing oil and this is important to remember. It protects against the loss of moisture and this is something quite different. It locks in the hair's natural moisture and retains its conditioning effect. So this is an oil that is beneficial to apply after the hair is fully conditioned and prior to any outdoor activity in which the hair would be subjected to pollution or extremes of heat, cold or wind.

This oil is not hard on the pocket and is easily available. It is an oil that is well worth having on hand and better still trying out.

It is important to note that there are many different types of Castor oil, many different grades, from therapeutic and cosmetic through to food-grade, household, medicinal, gardening, and manufacturing. The best types to use on the hair are the therapeutic or cosmetic grades and of the two, the therapeutic grade is preferable as it is free of harmful chemicals.

Always steer towards the best quality Castor oil and an organic brand if available. You should look for a clear, golden coloured oil that has a very mild and natural plant fragrance. This will be a good indication of quality.

Coconut Oil

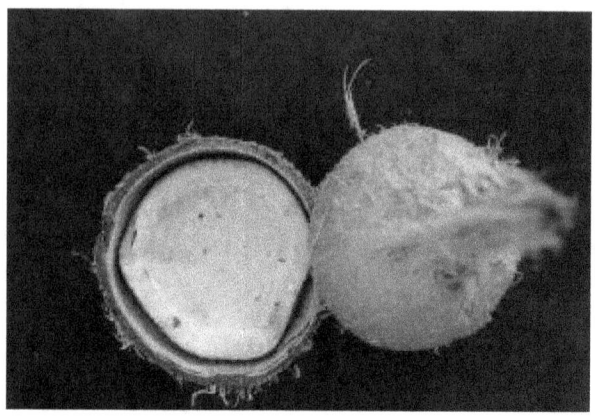

Photo Credit. Tiger Puppala. www.flickr.com/photos/puppala. Creative Commons

Coconut oil, which has often been dubbed 'the tree of life,' whether taken internally or used externally, has been proven to have many benefits.

It has dietary and other health benefits. Coconut oil has been studied quite extensively and shown to have wonderful properties that greatly enhance general hair health. This oil is known to penetrate the hair shaft with great efficiency and work its way through all the layers of a hair strand thereby moisturizing the hair shaft and replenishing proteins. This makes coconut oil an excellent hair conditioner and moisturizer, but this oil also helps to control dandruff and is effective in preventing hair fall.

For many decades we were warned against using coconut oil in our diets, but it has always retained its usefulness and popularity in Asian countries and recently, studies in the west show that actually instead of being detrimental to our health, coconut oil is quite the opposite, assisting in the health of the heart and helping to control many other diseases. Now, some are even calling it the 'Tree of Life' and it certainly lives up to this name.

It provides a nutritious source of milk, oil, and meat that feeds many people around the world. But aside from its amazing food value, coconut oil is also known for its wonderful medicinal properties. The list of its pro-ported benefits to health is a long one covering areas of vulnerability in all manner of bacterial, fungal and parasitic diseases to name but a few.

But getting back to coconut oil and its benefits for hair, we should mention a number of key components which are naturally present in this oil which makes it so useful for hair health.

Lauric Acid: An anti-microbial substance that acts upon the bacteria that are known to cause hair loss.

Capric Acid: Which is similar to Lauric Acid in that it is also anti-microbial, but it unites with the latter and increases its effectiveness.

Combining the above substances to its moisturizing and nutritive qualities one can understand why coconut oil is so highly valued by so many the world over.

When choosing a coconut oil it is wise to inspect the labels on products and choose one that is cold-pressed and therefore has had the minimum processing. This oil is easily and widely available as well as being very cost-effective. An excellent choice in hair care oils.

*****

Eucalyptus

Eucalyptus Oil comes from the Australian Blue Gum tree. The oil has a fresh and strident aroma and numerous medicinal properties.

Properties. Anti fungal, anti-microbial and anti-bacterial. Has bio-pesticide properties.

Benefits for Hair.

1. Effective in treating scalp conditions such as dandruff and psoriasis due to the presence of anti-fungal and anti-bacterial properties.

2. Encourages blood circulation if massaged into the scalp and is said to increase hair growth.

3. Moisturizes and soothes the hair follicles promoting a healthy scalp.

Side Effects. Eucalyptus oil should be used with care. It should never be taken internally and if used on the skin, should always be diluted with a carrier oil. Those with high blood pressure or epilepsy should avoid using it. In some people, it can also induce headaches.

*****

Evening Primrose Oil

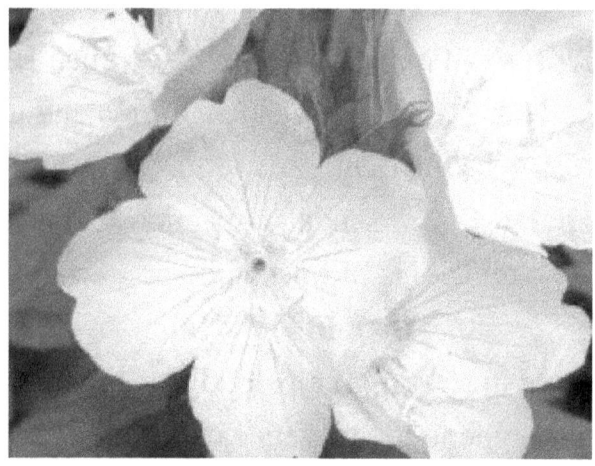

Photo Credit. H Bakkh. www.flickr.com/photos/8669065@N06. Creative Commons

Evening Primrose Oil is derived from the seeds of the Primrose Plant. The plant and the oil have many known medicinal uses but for our purposes, this oil is very beneficial and important as a natural treatment for skin and scalp disorders such as eczema and psoriasis.

This is an oil that is high in essential fatty acids, but it is primarily the fatty acid referred to as GLA that is responsible for much of its remarkable healing and prophylactic properties. Only a few other plants are known to contain such high quantities of this substance. Therefore, Evening Primrose Oil is a very important medicinal herb.

The boon for hair, with the use of this oil on a regular basis, or by way of adding some drops of it to a carrier oil, lies in its ability to absorb easily and quickly into the skin and hair shafts carrying the essential nutrients straight to where they are most needed. Massaging the oil into the scalp will also effectively relieve dandruff and other scalp conditions.

It might also be mentioned that Evening Primrose Oil is also considered an effective natural headache medicine. There are many beneficial qualities that make this oil a great choice for anyone with a known scalp condition and any of the problems associated with that.

This is a somewhat delicate oil and refrigeration is encouraged after the bottle has been opened. Its shelf life is approximately six to twelve months depending on how you store it.

There are no known contraindications from the use Evening Primrose oil, but as always, one should exercise caution if known allergies are present. Because this is such a fragile oil, go for cold-pressed brands where possible.

*****

Flaxseed Oil

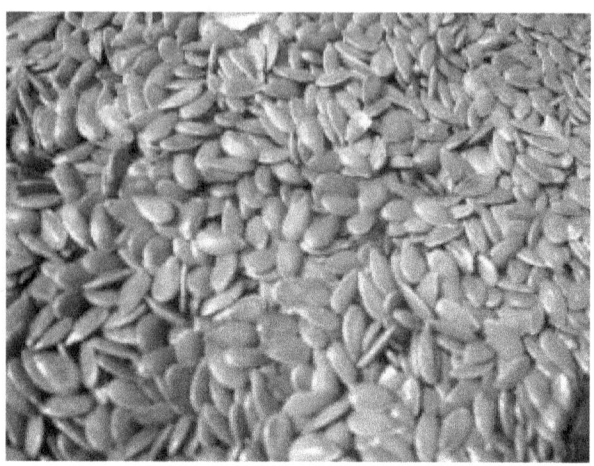

Photo Credit. Health Aliciousness. www.flickr.com/photos/healthaliciousness. Creative Commons

Flaxseed oil is a potent source of EFAs, (essential fatty acids) which we know are very useful for maintaining healthy skin and hair. Of the EFAs that are present in Flaxseed or Linseed as it is also known, linoleic acid is foremost.

However, this is not a stable oil and oxidizes within a few weeks of processing. This means that a cold-pressed oil should be refrigerated and as soon as the odour changes it should be discarded. This aspect of Flaxseed oil makes it somewhat challenging to market.

Flaxseed is known to be a rich source of omega 3 fatty acids which are effective in treating hair loss caused by stress and the damaging effects of stress on the whole immune system. It certainly does have an impressive nutrient value.

An interesting fact in relation to the EFAs in Flaxseed, and one that is likely to gain a good deal more attention in the future, is its ability to inhibit an enzyme that has an effect on the male hormone testosterone, and which is now thought to be a factor in the progression of balding and hair loss.

This is a reasonably priced oil but as mentioned above, the shelf life is very short at just a few weeks and must be refrigerated once opened. It does have some remarkable qualities however and is well worth investigating for oneself.

*****

Green Tea Seed Oil

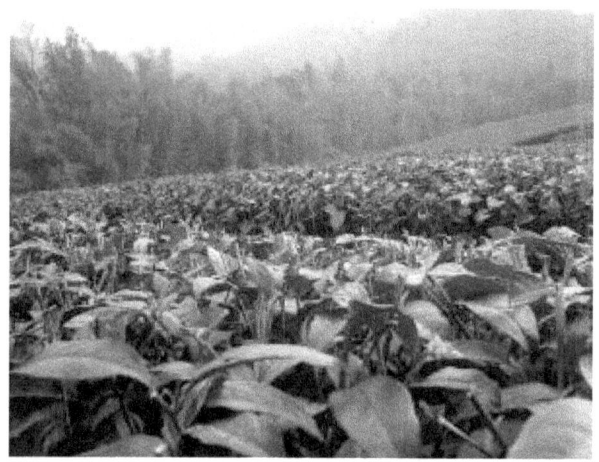

Photo Credit. Wm Jas. www.flickr.com/photos/healthaliciousness. Creative Commons

Green Tea Seed Oil has some unique and potent properties. It has been studied in Taiwan and the results show that this oil has anti-fungal, anti-bacterial and anti-septic properties, as well as some unique components such as saponins.

Saponins are naturally present in some food items such as legumes, spinach, alfalfa, and ginseng and of course Green Tea Seeds. They are phytochemicals that foam up when shaken inside water. Briefly, they are known to have various health benefits from lipid-lowering to cancer cell inhibition and boosting the immune system.

As all the health benefits associated with ingesting this oil are said also to be obtained from using it externally, one can understand that this is a very valuable resource with great health benefit potentials not only for hair!

This oil, which is derived from the seeds of the tea shrub called Camellia Sinensis, originated in China many centuries ago and was widely used as a culinary oil that has not only great nutritional value but also tastes really good.

Green Tea Seed oil has a greenish colour and a light and slightly tea leafy fragrance. It adds a very distinctive flavour to any dishes that are cooked with it.

However, the Chinese have also long recognized its medicinal properties, as well as its exceptional qualities as a moisturizer for both hair and skin.

Personally, I am very impressed with what I have been able to discover about it so far. Our skin and hair absorb nutrients and these are required to maintain their lustre and health and this is a process that goes on both internally and externally. So an oil that is both edible and also a great moisturizer has considerable value and potential for holistic use.

As previously mentioned all the benefits associated with drinking this tea are all present with the use of the oil.

The shelf life is approximately two years, so this is a stable oil and will retain its usefulness for a long period.

*****

Grape Seed Oil

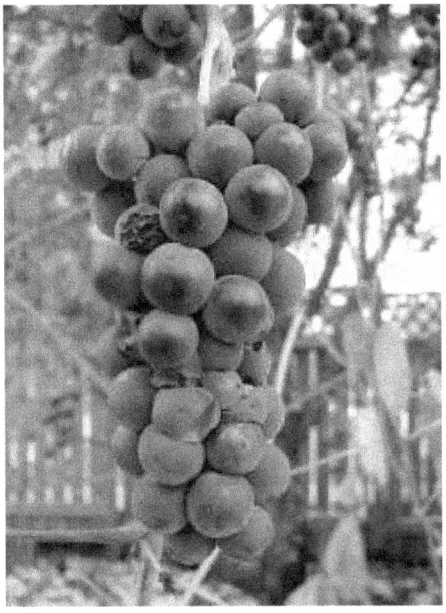

Photo Credit. Chris Campbell. www.flickr.com/photos/cgc. Creative Commons

Grape Seed Oil is extracted from the grape seeds after they have been used to make wine. It is a light oil and does not leave a greasy film on the hair or skin.

Properties. This is a polyunsaturated oil with a number of essential fatty acids such as linoleic acid. It contains a number of anti-oxidants, most notably Vitamin E along with minerals.

Benefits for Hair. Grape seed oil has numerous benefits for skin and hair care.

1. It adds lustre to the hair.

2. If massaged regularly into the scalp it will help relieve and slowly eliminate dandruff problems.

3. It protects the hair from harsh environmental conditions, sealing in the hairs natural moisture.

4. High levels of linoleic acid make it an excellent moisturizer and hair food.

5. If you have dry hair that tends to frizz after washing, this oil is a great choice in helping to tame the frizz.

6. If one has dyed or tinted hair, this oil will act as a great restorative.

7. A very useful oil for hot oil hair treatments.

8. It has natural anti-inflammatory properties that make it a useful treatment for scalp conditions such as psoriasis.

Other Uses. Grape seed oil is an excellent cooking oil. It's certainly up there with the best of them, namely coconut oil and olive oil. It has a very high smoking point and heat threshold which is excellent for culinary use.

Things to Look Out For. This oil is usually processed chemically, which makes the oil cheaper. The refined oil is normally stabilized with chemicals in order to increase its shelf life. It is **important** to note that two grades of Grape Seed oil are available on the market. One is for culinary use and the other is used in cosmetic and hair oil preparations. The one used in cosmetics is stabilized with a number of chemicals that should not be ingested.

If you intend to purchase this oil for use as a hair oil, go for an organic and cold-pressed brand. Take note of the colour. A greenish colour is desirable and indicative of less processing. After you open the bottle, be sure to store it in the fridge to maximize its shelf life.

Indications. There are a number of things to watch out for with the use of this oil. Those with known skin sensitivity and allergies should exercise caution when using the oil. If it is used in cooking, it may interfere with the use of anti-coagulants and medicines that lower cholesterol. These kinds of reactions are likely only to take place after prolonged use but this should nevertheless be kept in mind.

*****

Hemp Seed Oil

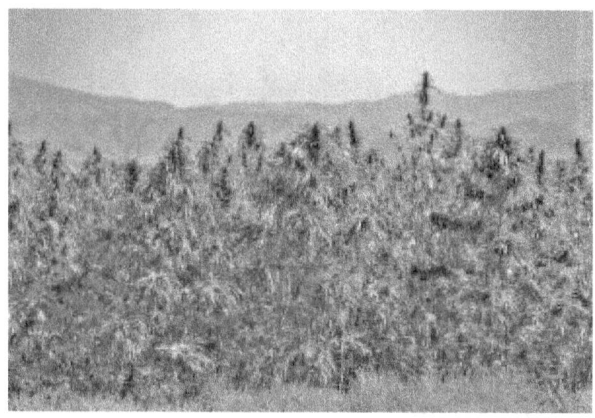

Photo Credit. Gregory Jordan. www.flickr.com/photos/gregoryjordan. Creative Commons

Hemp Seed Oil has many benefits for the hair. This oil is a truly nutrient-rich and very promising hair oil. It is loaded with essential fatty acids that play a big part in maintaining the elasticity of both hair and skin.

As the name suggests, Hemp seed oil is derived from the seeds of the hemp plant. Although the refined product is colourless and flavourless, in its organic and cold-pressed form, it is a clear and dark green oil with a pleasant nutty fragrance. If the oil has a darker colour it will also have a stronger flavour and smell and the organic, cold-pressed oil will retain its nutrients and be of far greater use for the hair.

If one is looking for a hair oil that promotes optimum health and sheen, the regular use of Hemp Seed oil will go a long way toward achieving this end. In particular, people with hair that is on the thicker side and more curly can use this oil, not only to tame the tangle and tone down the frizz, but it will nourish and protect the hair from excess breakage, which is an ongoing issue for curly hair types.

Virgin cold-pressed oil appears to have a brief shelf life. This is due to its high concentration of unsaturated fatty acids. This is somewhat countered in the refined version but then one loses much of the nutrient value of the oil during the processing. It would seem that once opened, refrigeration is advisable, just as is the case with Flaxseed oil.

Hemp Seed Oil has a very high percentage of essential fatty acids, along with numerous other nutrients. As a culinary oil, the organic version has a low heating threshold and therefore is not suitable for all types of cooking. However, its value as an external moisturizing oil for both hair and skin is becoming ever more recognized and appreciated.

This is an oil to look out for and no doubt one that people will begin to notice more and more in the future. It deserves the attention.

Horse Chestnut Oil

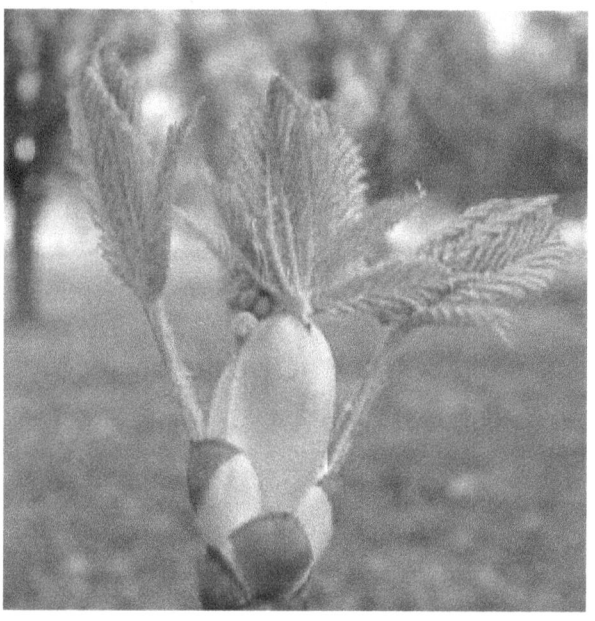

Photo Credit. Another Photograph. www.flickr.com/photos/anotherphotograph. Creative Commons

Horse Chestnut Oil is derived from the Horse Chestnut Tree which is also known by the name of Conker Tree.

Properties. The oil has many anti-oxidants. It is said to have anti-inflammatory and anti-rheumatic properties and is rich in essential fatty acids.

Benefits for Hair.

1. This oil helps to protect skin and hair from the damaging effects of UV rays.

2. It is a nourishing oil.

3. The oil has anti-inflammatory properties which make it useful in the treatment of scalp conditions such as dandruff and psoriasis. Also effective again dry, flaky scalp and itchiness.

4. It an effective moisturizer and conditioner.

5. Hydrates the skin and hair assisting in elasticity and prevents further drying out.

6. It is an emollient that also assists in preventing further damage to weakened hair.

Shelf Life. It has been noted that this oil will last up to three years if properly stored, but when macerated with other oils this shelf life may vary. Always refer to the expiration date on the label of any products you purchase.

Side Effects. There are indications that make this oil **unsuitable** for use where the skin has been broken or ulcerated. Horse Chestnut oil contains poisonous substances and care is required with its use where the above conditions are noted. There should also be caution where known allergies are present.

****

Hibiscus Flower Oil

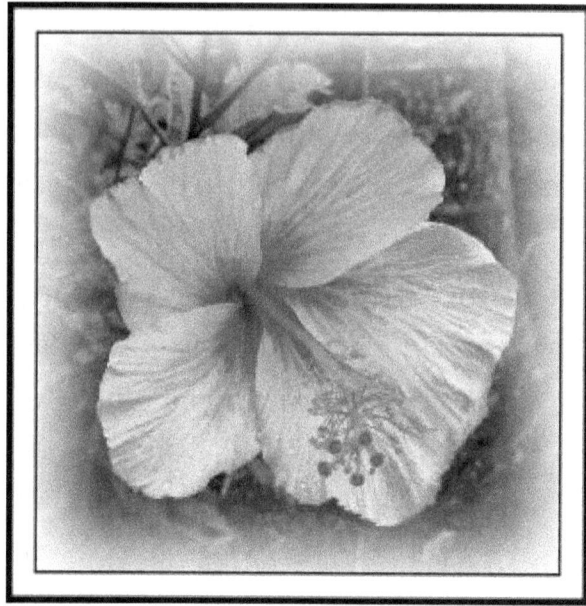

Photo Credit. Moments for Zen. www.flickr.com/photos/momentsforzen. Creative Commons.

Hibiscus Flower Oil combines a number of useful properties which are beneficial for hair care.

There are known to be over 200 different species of Hibiscus and most of these are used for their medicinal properties in Natural, Chinese and Indian Ayurveda medicines and herbal treatments.

It is often used in Ayurvedic Hair oil preparations because it is known to stimulate the hair follicles and therefore enhance hair growth. Where there is hair loss this oil will help to stop the hair fall and also slow down the greying process.

It is an effective oil in the treatment of scalp conditions such as dandruff and dry scalp. Its nutrient combinations make it easy to absorb into the hair and skin and as this is a rich oil it not only moisturizes the hair but also effectively helps to restore weakened and damaged hair to a stronger and more healthy condition.

It is also known for its ability to enhance natural as well as dyed hair colouring, adding lustre and sheen, while also sealing and protecting the hair. This is why it is often used in shampoos and conditioners.

Hibiscus oil also contains anti-inflammatory properties as well as being astringent. This is certainly an oil that has many useful benefits for hair.

It has a light and pleasant fragrance and is a very reasonably priced hair oil that has a good shelf life of at least one year.

*****

Jojoba Oil

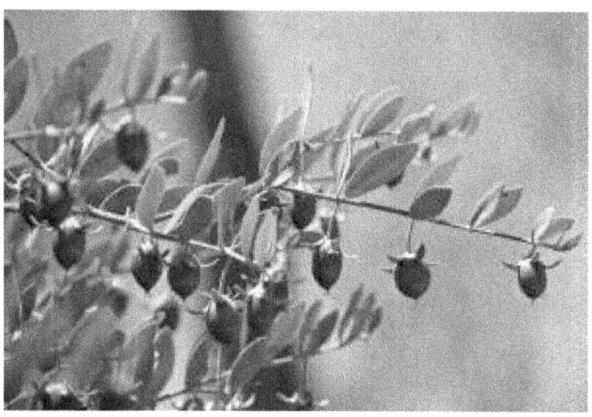

Photo Credit. Kretyen. www.flickr.com/photos/kretyen. Creative Commons

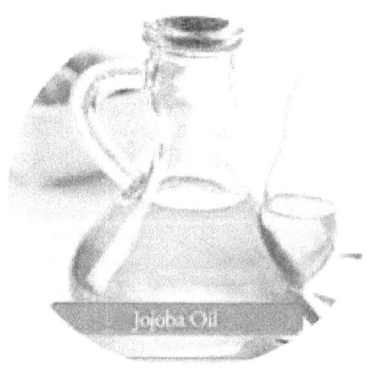

Jojoba oil is the lightest natural oil available on the market today. It is non-greasy and penetrates the skin and hair follicles with great ease.

Its 'lightness' makes it the most easily absorbed hair oil giving a weightless shine and lustre to the hair.

Jojoba is a small evergreen shrub that grows in the desert areas of the southwest USA and northwest Mexico. This small tree produces single seed fruits from which the oil is extracted. In these areas, it has long been known and appreciated for its wonderful healing properties.

Interestingly it is actually composed of liquid wax esters rather than oil. We find that the body's natural sebum also contains these same wax esters. These act as a natural moisturizer and protection for skin and hair shafts, but with age, their production decreases.

The wonderful natural properties of Jojoba, so closely resembles natural sebum, making it an ideal oil, not only for skin but also for hair. It has a balancing effect on the sebum production of our bodies preventing it from becoming too oily or too dry.

This oil contains many important nutrients such as Vitamins E and B complex, minerals such as silicon, zinc and also an abundance of natural iodine which gives it anti-bacterial and anti-fungal properties. All these properties have a combined effect on the hair which is beneficial for, not only conditioning the hair but also in treating a number of scalp conditions such as dandruff and psoriasis. It is also believed that Jojoba has a beneficial effect in preventing hair loss.

This makes it a valuable hair care product with a broad usefulness.

If you are considering buying this product, always try to buy a brand which is labelled 'cold pressed' or 'expeller pressed'. These manufacturing processes use less heating and subsequently, cause less damage to the natural product. One should also look for an oil which is light golden in colour and which has retained a light fragrance, both of which indicate purity and freshness.

There is no doubt that Jojoba oil is an important and very beneficial addition to hair oil products.

*****

Kiwi Seed Oil, the Chinese Gooseberry

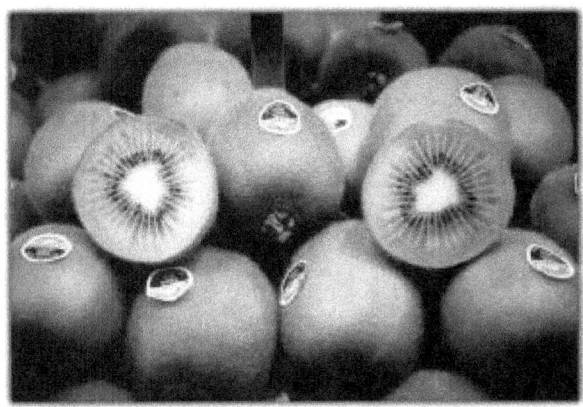

Photo Credit. Moyan Brenn. www.flickr.com/photos/aigle_dore. Creative Commons

Kiwi Seed Oil is derived, as the name suggests, from the seeds of the Kiwi Fruit which are also known by the name of Chinese Gooseberries. Kiwi Fruit has been cultivated in New Zealand for the past sixty years but originated in Asia.

Kiwi Fruit is particularly rich in Vitamin C and is second only to Guava for nutrient richness. The oil from the seeds of this fruit is also a rich source of essential fatty acids and alpha-linoleic acids along with other EFAs and AFAs.

A special process to separate the tiny and delicate seeds of the Kiwi Fruit from the pulp has been developed in New

Zealand. After this has taken place, the seeds are stabilized and processed.

The good news for skin and hair is in this oil's rich and concentrated levels of EFA, and AFA, both of which are crucial and valuable additions to skin and hair care products.

Kiwi Seed Oil if used alone provides a great and intensive conditioning and moisturizing treatment for the hair and skin. It is useful in the treatment of skin conditions such as acne and is also very effective in the treatment of scalp conditions such as dandruff and psoriasis. It does not clog the pores but rather assists in balancing skin and scalp oil production and thereby promotes the growth of healthy hair and skin.

It is widely used in anti-aging creams due to its high anti-oxidant properties and is also said to lighten dark skin areas under the eyes.

The health benefits of this oil, when used both internally and externally, are considerable.

Cold-pressed Kiwi Seed Oil has a shelf life of approximately two years if properly stored. There are no reported contraindications for the use of this oil and unless one has known allergies, it can be used safely.

This is a multi-purpose oil and one that bestows considerable benefits for skin and hair.

Kukui Seed Oil

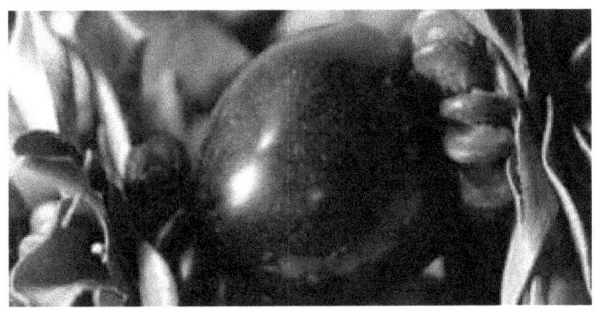

Photo Credit. Hawaii Kukui Nut Oil. www.hawaiiikukuinutoil.com.

Kukui Nut Oil is derived from the seeds of the Kukui Nut Tree which is the State Tree of Hawaii. This tree also goes by the name of the Candlenut Tree. The oil from the Kukui Nut has long been used by the locals to protect their skin from the drying effects of heat and salt from the ocean. These days it is used in many skin and hair care products that are now being produced in the West.

Properties. This oil is rich in essential fatty acids, Vitamins, and minerals.

Benefits for Hair.

1. It is an excellent emollient oil.

2. Conditions and moisturizes the hair.

3. Adds shine and lustre to the hair.

4. Protects the hair from harsh environmental factors.

5. Helps to regenerate and restore damaged and broken hair.

Shelf Life. There seem to be two sets of thought about the shelf life of Kukui Nut oil. One claims that it has a shelf life of six to eight months while the other school of thought indicates that it has a much longer life of approximately two years. I am sure that the way the oil is stored would play a large part in which one is correct.

Side Effects. There are no noted contraindications with the use of this oil but if known sensitivity and allergies are present, caution is advised.

*****

Lavender Oil

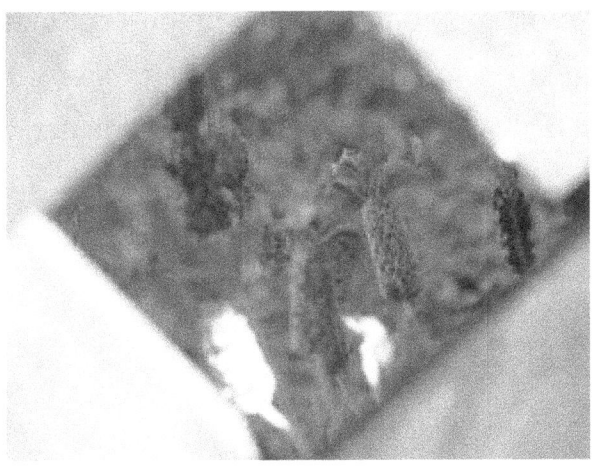

Photo Credit. Hicky Scott. www.flickr.com/photos/hickey-scott. Creative Commons

Lavender Oil is an aromatic and tonic essential oil with a sweet fragrance. It has many medicinal uses and is also a favourite in aromatherapy.

Benefits for Hair. It has a number of beneficial uses for hair, treating various hair and scalp conditions.

1. Very effective in the treatment of hair loss.

2. Used to treat dry scalp.

3. Dandruff and psoriasis are also said to respond well to the regular use of this essential oil.

4. It has a calming and soothing effect when rubbed into the scalp assisting with conditions such as stress and insomnia.

5. Significantly enhances the blood's circulation to the scalp thereby promoting increased hair growth.

Side Effects. As with essential oils in general, Lavender oil should not be taken internally and where allergies are known, caution is advised.

*****

Lemon Oil

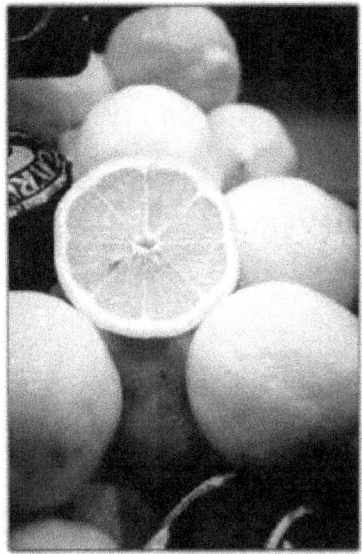

Photo Credit. Moya Brenn. www.flickr.com/photos/aigle_dore. Creative Commons

Lemon Oil is one of the foremost foods when it comes to the content of both minerals and vitamins. The oil is extracted from the lemon rind and has been in use since Roman times when it was applied to ward off insects and keep bugs from eating fabrics.

Properties. It has a high anti-oxidant content and is an anti-fungal, antiseptic, anti-bacterial and anti-inflammatory.

This is by no means an exhaustive list of its medicinal benefits.

Benefits for Hair.

1. A great cleansing and astringent oil.
2. Has a nourishing effect on the hair.
3. Assists in the treatment of scalp conditions such as dandruff and psoriasis.
4. Helps in cleansing the scalp of sebum deposits.
5. Has a stimulating effect on the hair roots and follicles which in turn assists in healthy hair growth.
6. Soothes irritating scalp conditions by clearing away build-up.
7. Helpful in conditions of dry or oily scalp helps to balance the scalp oils natural production.

Side Effects. Lemon oil should not be used directly on the skin as this may cause irritation, so dilute it before applying. Where known allergies are present, caution is advised.

*****

Mango Oil

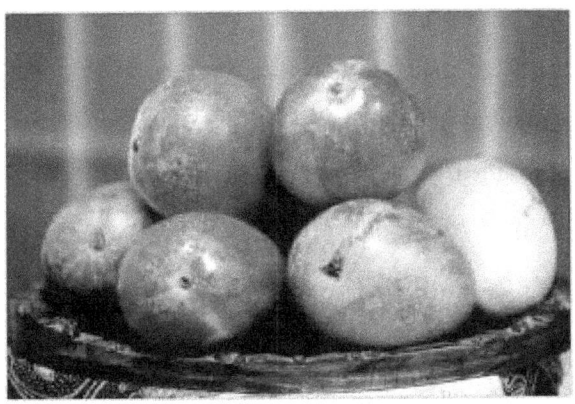

Photo Credit. Dihlie. www.flickr.com/photos/dihlie. Creative Commons

Mango Oil is derived from the seed of the Mango fruit. It is semi-solid at room temperature but melts upon contact with the skin making it a good oil for use in cosmetic preparations.

Properties. Rich in essential fatty acids and anti-oxidants.

Benefits for hair.

1. An emollient that protects against harsh environmental extremes of heat, cold, wind and dry.

2. Mango Oil also protects weakened and damaged hair against further splitting and drying.

3. A great softener and conditioner of both skin and hair.

4. Moisturizes and nourishes.

5. Rehydrates the hair while also nourishing it with its numerous anti-oxidants.

6. Helps to regenerate the hair when it is in a weakened condition, restoring elasticity and shine.

Shelf Life. Mango oil has an impressively long shelf life of three to four years with proper storage.

Side Effects. Caution is advised where known allergies are present.

*****

Meadowfoam Oil

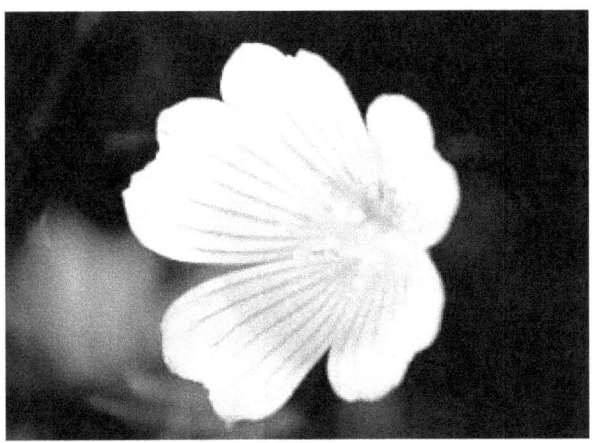

Photo Credit. David Hoffman. www.flickr.com/photos/23326361@N04. Creative Commons

Meadowfoam Oil is derived from the seeds of the Meadowfoam plant, a native of northern California, southern Oregon, and British Columbia. This oil is unique for its stability and a number of other factors.

There is an impressive list of properties pertaining to Meadowfoam oil namely;

1. It contains over 98% long-chain fatty acids.

2. It has high-grade triglyceride levels.

3. It contains three long-chain fatty acids that were unknown to science prior to their discovery of the oil of this plant's seeds.

All of this is good news for your hair and skin. Meadowfoam oil is used in many cosmetic and hair products due to its numerous properties. It has also been found that by adding it to other less stable oils it will extend their shelf life too.

Meadowfoam is an oil that is a wonderful conditioner and moisturizer. It is both light and easily absorbed and does not leave greasy or filmy traces behind on the skin or hair. It is nutrient-rich and has powerful regenerative properties that protect as well as help to restore hair and skin alike.

Although Meadowfoam seeds are fed to cattle, the oil is not used for cooking or eaten by humans. Its uses at this stage are purely external and mostly for cosmetics and hair products, although it is currently being studied to gauge its wider uses.

As previously mentioned it has a long and stable shelf life.

*****

Maracuja Oil

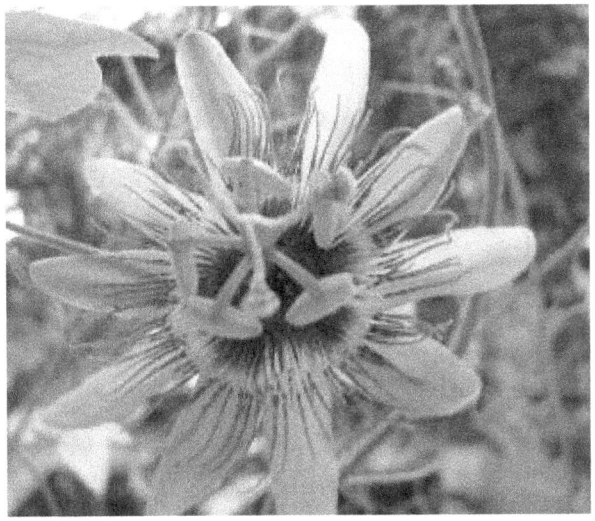

Maracuja Oil, also known as Passion Fruit Seed Oil (Passiflora Incarnata) is a high-quality emollient as well as being a nutrient-rich oil.

Maracuja or Passionflower Oil is packed with essential fatty acids, in particular, linoleic acid which is present in a high concentration of some 70% and oleic acid at around 12%. These two EFAs are very important when it comes to skin and hair care. Aside from these two fatty acids, the oil also contains stearic and palmitic acids in lesser concentrations.

Maracuja has a reasonable shelf life of between one and two years and is produced by both cold-pressing extraction methods and as a refined oil. We generally prefer the organic and cold-pressed oils because they retain more of their natural nutrients.

Its benefits for hair and skin are numerous;

1. High-quality emollient.

2. Conditioner, moisturizer for both hair and skin. It does not leave any greasy traces on the skin or hair and is a light oil that can be used on all hair types.

3. Helps to repair dry, damaged and weakened hair and skin.

4. Is a potent nourishing oil with high absorption properties and very importantly, it does not clog the pores of the skin but just absorbs easily and smoothly.

5. The oil has anti-inflammatory and also anti-microbial properties making it a useful oil for treating scalp conditions such as dandruff and psoriasis and dry scaly scalp.

The list goes on. Although Maracuja originated in the rainforests of the Amazon it has spread far and wide and now grows throughout much of Asia and north and south America.

This oil is a valuable addition to hair care oils and its regular use greatly improves the overall health of both hair and skin, restoring its lustre and giving it a new lease of life.

*****

Macadamia Oil, A Boon For Dry Hair

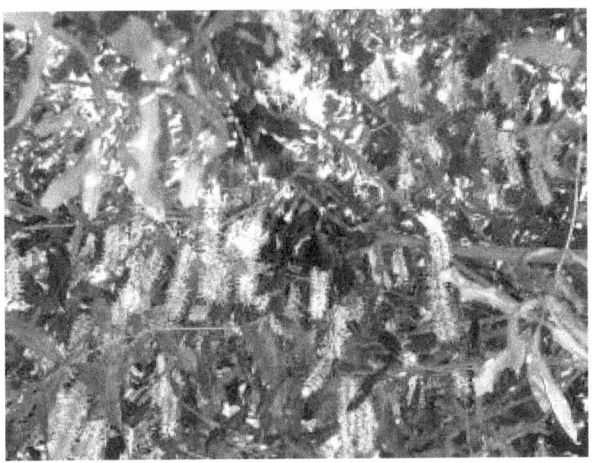

Photo Credit. Wiccked. www.flickr.com/photos/wiccked. Creative Commons

Macadamia oil is derived from the macadamia nut. This is a lightweight oil with high nutrient values. Its molecular composition bares a strong resemblance to the natural sebum of the scalp. This affinity makes it a very effective moisturizer with rapid absorption levels and effective assimilation.

The component that sets this oil apart from many of the others is its high concentration of palmitic acid. Because this is also found in human sebum it is a valuable natural nutrient-rich oil that has many benefits for hair.

It is no exaggeration to say that Macadamia oil is a boon for hair and skin. If one uses this oil on a regular basis, results are not long in the coming. It works its magic swiftly and replaces moisture. It is an effective emollient sealing moisture into the hair shaft, thereby not only rehydrating the hair but also protecting it from further damage.

It is said to restore damaged and weakened hair, add lustre, shine and also to protect and shield from chemicals and pollutants in the environment. It is also effective in blocking UV rays.

So as you can see from the above information this is a valuable addition to hair oil treatments and likely to increase significantly in popularity as people become aware of just how useful and effective this oil can be.

As a hair oil one should look for an organic brand that has used a cold-pressing method for processing.

Macadamia oil has a twenty-month shelf life, which is another advantage with this oil

Monoi Oil

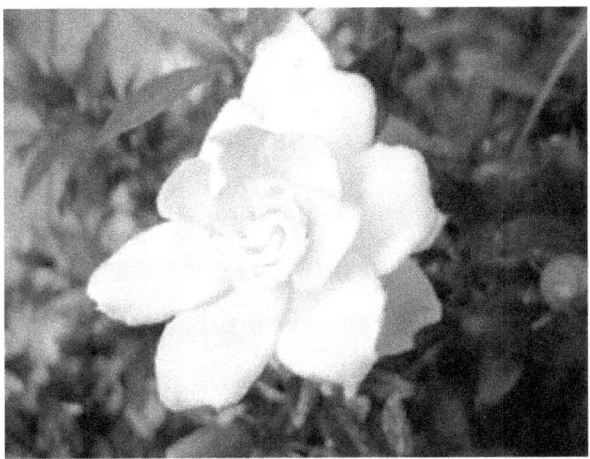

Photo Credit. Ma Zoa Arts. www.flickr.com/photos/jlmbewe. Creative Commons

Monoi Oil originated in the South Pacific Islands some 2000 years ago, its history inextricably linked to the lives of the Maoris. But it was not until the 1760 s, when Captian Cook stumbled across its use among the tribes living on some of the islands which he visited, that it came to be known to Europeans.

Monoi oil is produced by soaking the petals of gardenias in semi-waxed coconut oil. This infusion is used primarily on the skin and hair but also covers many other purposes in the lives of these people from their birthright up until their deaths.

Monoi which means 'scented oil' is used to anoint newborns and is also used to embalm the dead. Some of its medicinal uses range from the treatment of headaches to the relief of sunburn. The islanders of the South Pacific would coat themselves in this oil before undertaking long sea journeys as it was known to help protect their skin from the effects of prolonged exposure to seawater and the sun. Even today divers apply Monoi oil before making dives as it helps the body to retain its heat.

For the hair, Monoi oil is primarily useful as a conditioner and it also adds a coating that helps to protect the hair from harsh climatic extremes of heat and cold, sun and rain. However, it also has a very pleasant natural scent, thanks to the Gardenias and this makes it a great leave-in hair oil that is multifunctional.

Monoi is more than 90 per cent coconut oil which, after a careful process of milling, crushing, pressing and finally filtering is stabilized with the addition of vitamin E. After this, the petals from the gardenias are added to the oil. When it is carried out properly, 10 buds of gardenias per litre of oil must be soaked for a period not less than two weeks.

This is one oil that has been subjected to careful and well-documented research and so its many purported benefits are not just the imaginings of the locals. According to the www.monoi-institute.org, a research institute based in Tahiti, this oil is a nutrient-rich moisturizer that continues to work on the skin and hair for many hours together.

If you have an outdoor lifestyle and enjoy sports and travel this could well be an oil to consider trying.

Although many prototypes of Monoi oil are available on the market today, the genuine article is carefully produced and accredited. The island of Tahiti in French Polynesia is a major producer of this oil today. It even has a special provision written into a government seal to ensure quality and authenticity. So if you want to be certain of the quality you are buying you should keep this in mind and search out brands that have the proper authentication.

There are several small Tahitian enterprises that are producing this oil as a quality product and following the traditional methods. The oldest and perhaps the best known among these is a company called The Parfumerie Tiki.

*****

Moringa Oil

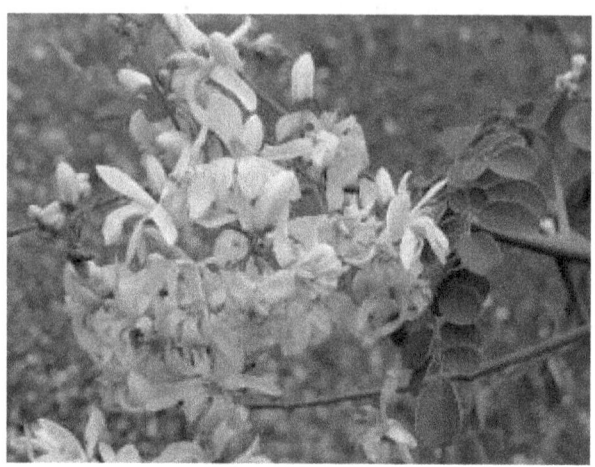

The **Moringa** Oleifera Tree grows in the Himalayas but is widely cultivated throughout India. It is purported to be one of the most nutritious plants on the planet. It contains an impressive number of anti-oxidants which take it into a category of its own not only as an edible plant but also as a nutrient-rich oil in the world of skincare and beauty products.

However, this plant has a long history and has been used and appreciated since the time of the Egyptians who buried vials containing the precious oil in their tombs. Moringa oil is widely used throughout the Middle Eastern and South Asian countries. In fact, the drumsticks, which are the immature seed pods of the tree have shown up in many a traditional meal that I have eaten, particularly in the South of India.

The oil from this tree is extracted from its seeds. Because of its very high potencies of anti-oxidants, it has a natural preservative effect on the oil helping it to retain its quality and goodness many years after it has been extracted from the seeds. This is another factor that enhances its attractiveness in the use of cosmetics.

It is highly prized in the composition of skincare products, in particular, those meant as anti-ageing potions with a 70+% oleic acid which greatly enhances skin and hair absorption carrying nutrients quickly and easily to the cells. It also blends easily with essential oils which can add extra effectiveness to any oil as a whole.

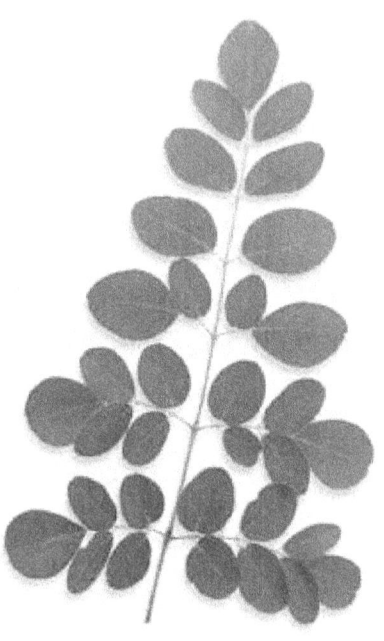

As a hair care oil, it can be used on the hair as a complete hair care treatment and when massaged into the scalp the effects of regular use are quickly apparent. It has not been called 'hair food' without good reason.

Moringa oil is suitable for all skin and hair types so it has a potentially vast reach in terms of usability. This is an oil to look out for.

*****

Mongongo Oil

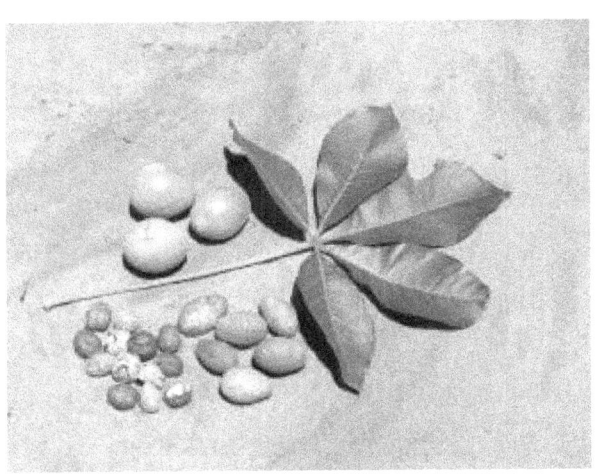

Mongongo Oil is derived from the kernels of the fruit of the Mongongo Tree which grows throughout much of Africa. The fruits of this tree are widely eaten by people and animals. In particular, the Elephant and Kudu, both of which feast on the fruits and then pass the nuts in their stools. These nuts are later collected and from them is produced the Mongongo Oil.

Properties. Mongongo oil has many essential fatty acids, in particular, it is said to contain a large amount of linoleic acid which is well known to have regenerating and hydration properties. It is also used to help in the restoration of weakened and damaged hair. The nutritional content of the kernels is as follows.

1. Polyunsaturated fatty acids - 43%
2. Monounsaturated fatty acids - 18%
3. Fats - 57%
4. Saturated fats - 17 %
5. Minerals.

Benefits for Hair. This is an oil that has multiple benefits for the hair from moisturizing and conditioning, protecting against UV rays, adding shine and lustre to repairing damaged hair ends. With such a list of benefits, this oil is bound to gain prominence in the world of hair oils. The numerous fatty acids in Mongongo oil make it a very nourishing hair oil and because it also contains large amounts of the Vitamin E, it is stable and has a long shelf life.

Marula Oil

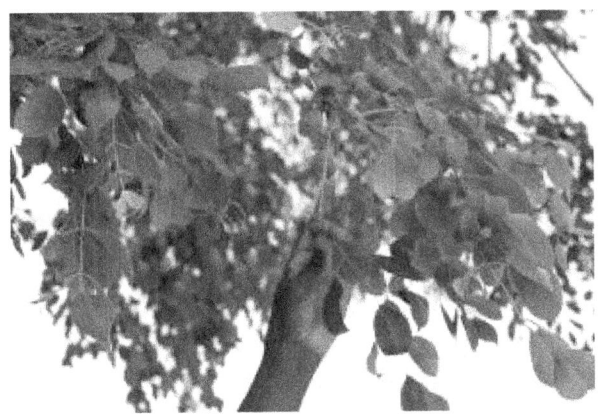

Photo Credit. Programme for Forest. www.flickr.com/photos/forestideas. Creative Commons

The **Marula** Tree grows in Mozambique and South Africa and has some interesting effects on the skin. It is known to reduce redness and pigmentation of the skin. Another effect of this oil is to help reduce epidermal water loss and is effective in skincare and tissue healing.

The Marula Oil has been known and used by African woman for many centuries and is widely valued for its moisturizing properties and its effects on creating more supple and less wrinkled skin. In a dry climate, this oil has very effective re-hydration properties.

This would have to be one of the great skin hydration oils available today. It is made up of mainly oleic acid but also contains palmitic and stearic acids and has a very light quality making it easy for the skin and hair shafts to absorb. Although primarily known as a great skin oil, there can be no doubt that Marula oil is also very valuable as an oil for hair. With a high absorption rate and unique combination of fatty acids, this oil contains properties that will benefit hair and greatly assist in its lustre and health.

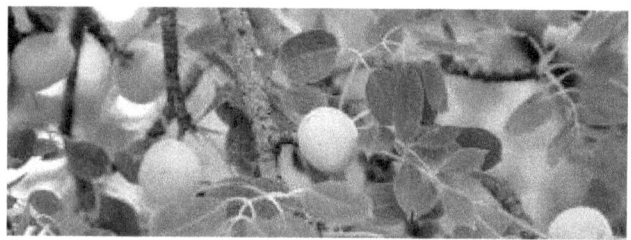

This is a light oil and absorbs easily and quickly when worked into the scalp and hair. Because Marula is a nutrient-rich oil it will strengthen weakened or damaged hair and help to maintain and protect healthy hair.

Marula oil has a long shelf life of approximately two years due to the high concentration of anti-oxidants within the oil.

This is proving to be a valuable resource for hair and skin and one that we are bound to hear more about in the West as time goes on.

*****

Myrtle Oil

Myrtle oil derived from the Myrtle bush which is a native of North Africa. This plant is very fragrant and grows to quite a large size.

Properties. Low concentrations of this oil are known to inhibit the growth of breast cancers and are second only to Sandalwood oil which has also been reported to have a similar effect. It has powerful astringent properties that are useful in balancing the condition of oily scalp.

Benefits for Hair.

1. This is an excellent oil for balancing and harmonizing the oils on the skin and scalp.
2. Assists in normalizing hormonal imbalances which in turn affect the natural sebum production of the scalp.
3. Has a calming effect when massaged into the scalp.
4. Has anti-bacterial properties which assist in treating scalp infections.
5. Has a soothing effect on the skin and scalp.

Side Effects. Myrtle oil, as with all essential oils, should be diluted before being applied directly to the skin and where known allergies are present, should be avoided or applied only after testing.

*****

Neem Oil

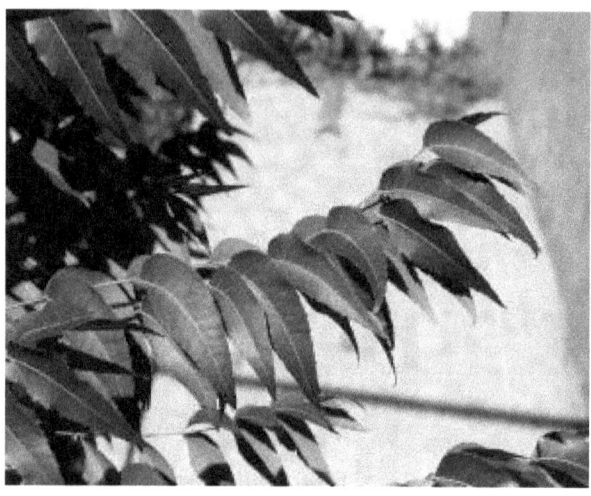

Photo Credit. Tatters. www.flickr.com/photos/tgerus. Creative Commons

I have come across Neem Oil very frequently in India. It is commonly used for a wide variety of different medical conditions but is also known and favoured for its ability to treat a number of hair conditions such as dandruff and dry or itchy scalp, dry hair and scalp infections. It is also known to treat head lice and nits.

In ancient Vedic times, the Neem tree was known as 'the cure for all illnesses' and it certainly deserves its important reputation as a healing oil. This is a multi-functional oil and one with particular benefits for hair care.

Neem oil is a thick oil and depending on how it is processed can look anything from golden to dark coloured. It has a not so pleasant odour, but as only a few drops are required and these are usually diluted in a carrier oil such as coconut or olive oil, the smell is not too much of a problem. But in this regard it might also be said, one can handle a 'little pain for much gain.'

Some evidence suggests that Neem has natural anti-microbial and anti-bacterial and anti-parasitic properties, which make it useful for scalp conditions such as psoriasis along with a whole host of other medical problems of a different nature.

Neem is also uniquely known to have concentrated levels of azadirachtin which is a natural form of insecticide. A compound found in Neem oil and the leaf extract, which is called Salannin is currently, being studied for its effective use as an insect repellent and it is important to note here that Neem is showing the promise of being even more effective than DEET and a whole lot safer!

Neem is a readily bio-degradable oil so it should be refrigerated. However, the cold-pressed, organic oil is said to have a shelf life of two years. I would advise refrigeration once opened and where possible.

Caution: this oil is only intended for external use and if it is in Essential and Concentrated oil form one should test a small area of skin prior to using it extensively.

*****

Olive Oil as a Carrier Oil for Hair

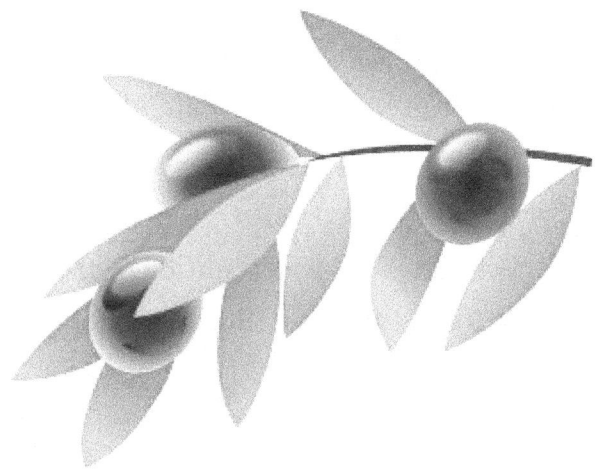

Olive oil is an excellent carrier oil for the hair. It has become such an integral part of our kitchens and our diets these days that we may not have ever known of or considered its importance as a 'carrier oil' for various hair oil treatments. Carrier oils are just that, they carry other oils or active ingredients onto the hair or skin. They provide a base for concentrated essential oils or medicinal tonics and unlike the latter, they do not evaporate. They have high absorption levels which assist the added medicinal or concentrated essences to be absorbed.

Pure virgin olive oil is easily available, not hard on the pocket, it is a great carrier oil that adds wonderful conditioning properties for the hair, has a long shelf life and on top of all of that, is packed full of nutrients in the form of minerals and vitamins which, because of its capacity to be easily absorbed, are readily assimilated by the hair shaft.

If you want to add essential oils in order to enhance treatments for either dryness, split ends, psoriasis, dandruff or whatever hair or scalp condition you may, by endeavouring to treat, this oil will provide an excellent and affordable base.

*****

Pine Nut Oil

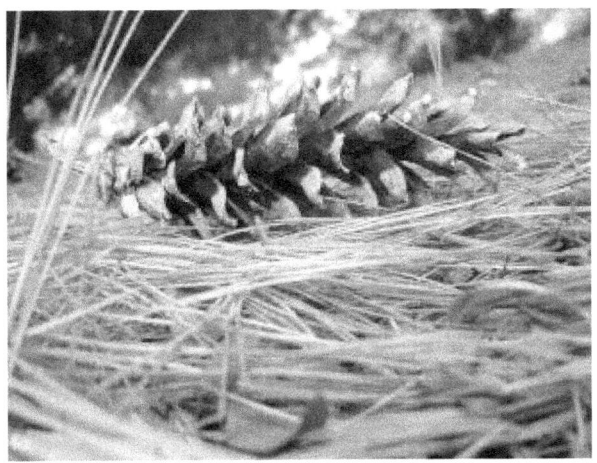

Photo Credit. Daily Dose of Joshy. www.flickr.com/photos/dailydoseofjoshy. Creative Commons

Pine Nut Oil is extracted from the seeds of a number of varieties of pine trees. The oil has uses both in the kitchen as a culinary oil and for external use.

Properties. The oil contains a high percentage of essential fatty acids and anti-oxidants. It also contains a fatty acid that is unique to the oil alone, namely that of pinolenic acid which is said to suppress the appetite and reduce bad cholesterol from building up in the arteries. Vitamins E and F are also prevalent in this oil and enhance its free radical scavenging effects.

Benefits for Hair.

1. Effective in treating scalp conditions such as dandruff and psoriasis.
2. Assist in the hydration and moisturizing of the hair.
3. Protects dry and brittle hair from further damage.
4. Nourishes the hair while also conditioning it.
5. It eliminates itching of the scalp.
6. Gives lustre and sheen to the hair.

Shelf Life. Has an approximately 12-month shelf life if properly stored.

Side Effects. There are no known side effects with the use of Pine Nut oil, but if known allergies are present caution should be exercised.

*****

Plum Seed Oil

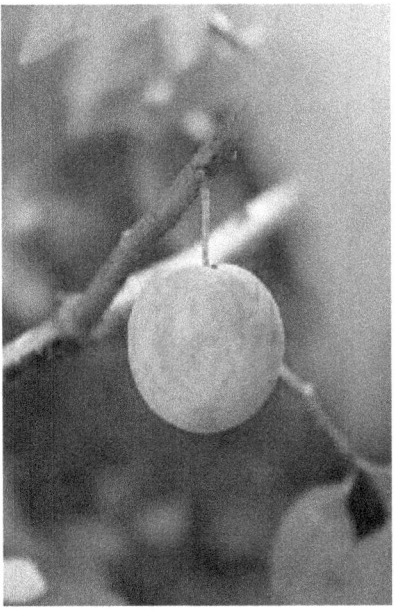

Photo Credit. Green Colander. www.flickr.com/photos/greencolander. Creative Commons

Plum Seed Oil is derived from dried plum pits and is also sometimes called Prune oil. It is a fine nutrient-rich oil with valuable applications for the cosmetic companies and a wide array of benefits for both skin and hair care.

Properties. Its nutrient profile is impressive. It contains a dense essential fatty acid profile and is also rich in fatty acids. This oil also has anti-oxidants in notable quantities, namely from the family of Tocopherols including, Alpha, Beta, Gamma and Delta Tocopherols

Benefits for Hair.

1. It has been shown to have a very marked ability to improve skin elasticity and nourish and protect the hair.

2. Absorbs quickly into the skin and hair without leaving greasy traces behind.

3. A highly effective moisturizer and conditioner.

4. Its high nutritive content makes it a valuable oil for weakened and damaged hair, as this oil assists in the nourishing and regeneration process.

5. An emollient oil.

6. Minimizes breakage due to dry and split hair ends.

7. Also noted for its effectiveness in the treatment of scalp conditions such as psoriasis.

This is a medium oil with a light golden colour and a fragrance that resembles that of Bitter Almond.

Shelf Life. Plum Seed oil is a stable oil with an approximate shelf life of two years if properly stored.

Side Effects. No known adverse effects from the external use of this oil. However, where known allergies are present caution should be exercised.

*****

Peach Kernel Oil

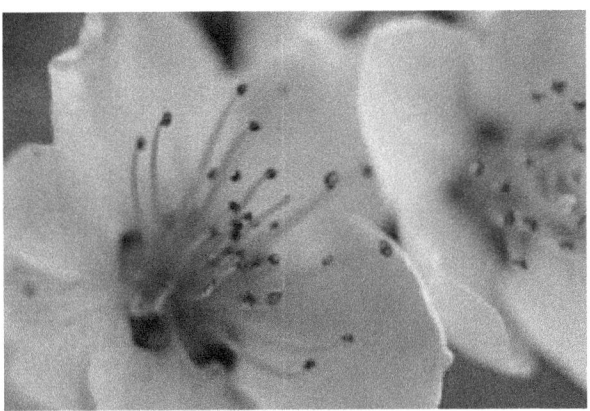

Photo Credit. Max Westby. www.flickr.com/photos/max_westby. Creative Commons

Peach Kernel Oil is a very useful carrier oil. This is a light and highly moisturizing oil and makes a great base to which essential oils can be added.

This oil is lighter than sweet almond and with a delicate and pleasant odour. It is a good moisturizing oil for people with slightly larger skin pores and somewhat ageing skin and assists in regenerating and moisturizing damaged and weakened hair.

This is a very safe carrier oil with no known hazards.

It contains a high percentage of Oleic acid, along with lesser amounts of all the other essential fatty acids. It is also said to contain high amounts of the Vitamins E and A and is, therefore, a nutrient-rich moisturizing oil.

Peach Kernel oil has approximately a one-year shelf life and as such is a relatively stable oil.

*****

Poppy Seed Oil

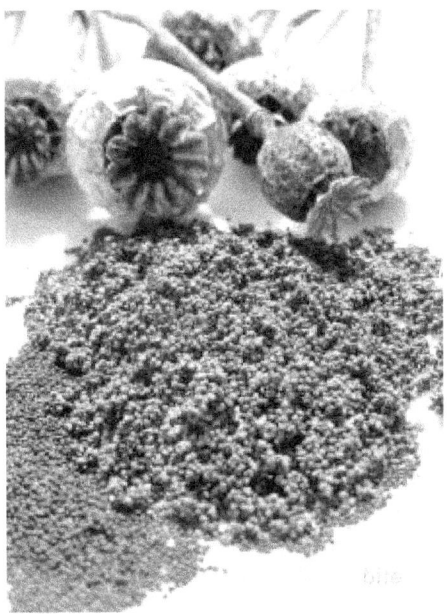

Photo Credit. Bite By Michele. http://bitebymichelle.com/2012/04/17/
citrus-glazed-poppy-seed-orange-and-lemon-muffins/april-16-2012-poppy-seed-muffins-034-cop.
Creative Commons

Poppy Seed oil is derived from one of the oldest cultivated plants in Europe. Today, however, it is a very popular carrier oil that is used widely by manufacturers in producing shampoos, conditioners and cosmetic preparations due to its moisturizing properties.

It is also popular for massage therapists and in aromatherapy treatments.

It makes an excellent carrier oil and has a long and stable shelf life.

Properties. Poppy Seed oil has a very nutrient-rich profile. The oil contains high levels of Vitamin E. It contains approximately 73% polyunsaturated fatty acids. 16% monounsaturated fatty acids. It contains high levels of linoleic acid, sometimes as high as 75% depending on how the oil is processed. The oil contains minerals and proteins Poppy Seed oil is colourless and odourless with some very similar properties to Safflower oil but with a few advantages over the latter.

The organic, cold-pressed and unrefined oil has a slightly different smell and texture, being nearer to the natural product it has retained more of its properties and nutrients, unlike the more highly refined oils that one can purchase in the supermarket.

Benefits for Hair.

1. Poppy Seed oil not only moisturizes the hair, but it also helps to smooth the hair cuticle which gives the hair a lovely sheen and lustre.

2. Conditions the hair and nourishes it.

3. Helps to regenerate and strengthen weakened or damaged hair.

4. Greatly enhances the appearance of the hair by adding shine and lustre.

5. Can also be used as a deep conditioning oil if left on the hair prior to shampooing

Shelf Life. Poppy Seed oil has a shelf life of approximately one year if properly stored.

Side Effects. Although thought to be entirely free of the side effects that are active when using other parts of this plant, Poppy Seed oil is not noted to contain any such adverse effects. However, where known allergies are present, caution is advised.

*****

Pistachio Nut Oil

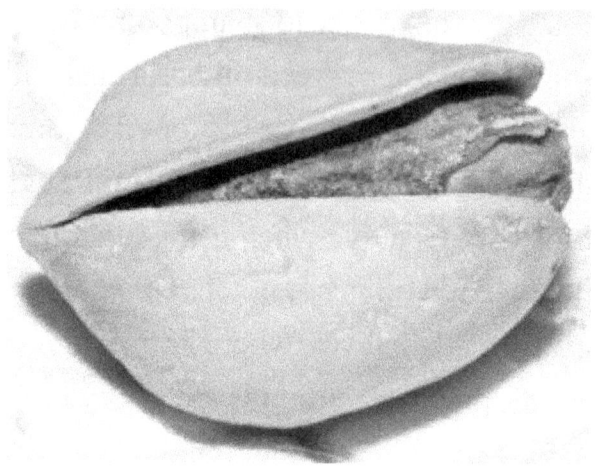

Photo Credit. Dave Dehetre. www.flickr.com/photos/davedehetre. Creative Commons

Pistachio Nut Oil is not only a delicious nut to eat but is packed with nutrition and goodness.

Properties. The oil has a high content of mono-unsaturated fatty acids. It also contains many anti-oxidants, namely Vitamins A and E and B Complex, as a well as a number of minerals such as copper and zinc. The oil is also rich in phytosterols which may have anti-cancer properties.

Benefits for Hair.

1. This is an emollient oil with great moisturizing properties.

2. Conditions and moisturizes the hair.

3. Protects against environmental extremes such as wind, heat, cold and dryness.

4. Is a very nourishing hair oil.

Shelf Life Pistachio Nut oil has a shelf life of approximately six months to one year and should be stored in the fridge after opening.

Side Effects. The nuts are known to cause allergic reactions in some people and although this is not likely to be a problem when using the oil externally, caution should be exercised when allergies are known to exist.

*****

Pecan Nut Oil

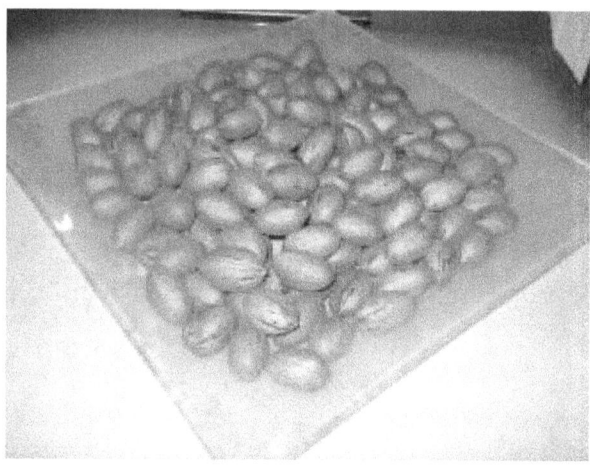

Photo Credit. Yale Berri. www.flickr.com/photos/yaelbeer. Creative Commons

Pecan Nut Oil is derived from the fruit of the Pecan tree which originated in North America but is now being cultivated as a valuable cash crop internationally. The Pecan tree is a branch of the Hickory family.

Properties The nuts are very nutrient-rich, containing a high percentage of monounsaturated fatty acids. They also contain a number of anti-oxidants, particularly Vitamins E, A and lutein. The nuts contain high levels of the Vitamins B complex along with a number of minerals such as magnesium, calcium, and iron.

Benefits for Hair

1. An effective conditioning and moisturizing oil.

2. Assists in the rehydration of hair and skin.

3. Emollient giving protection from harsh environmental extremes and protecting weakened or damaged hair from further breakage and splitting.

4. A very broad-based nutrient-rich hair oil that will nourish and condition at the same time.

5. Adds lustre and sheen to the hair.

Shelf Life This oil has a relatively short shelf life of approximately 6 months to one year. It should be kept in the fridge after opening.

Side Effects There is a type 1 hypersensitivity allergy response in some people from the use of this nut/oil. Where known allergies exist it may be better to avoid the use of this oil until testing has been done.

*****

Pomegranate Seed Oil

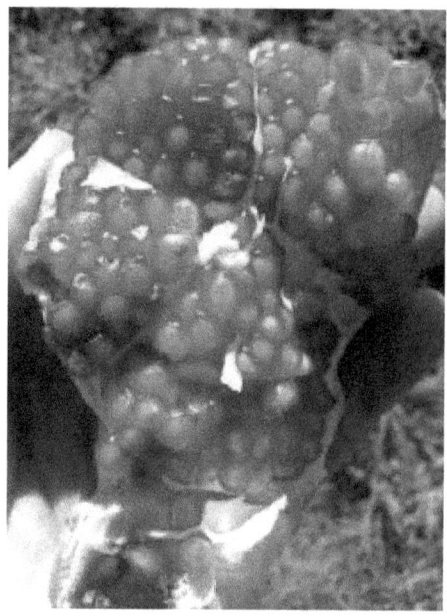

Photo Credit. MRPBPS. www.flickr.com/photos/mrpbps. Creative Commons

Pomegranate Seed Oil is a very effective oil when it comes to being used as a hair oil.

It has a beautiful soft amber colour and a slightly tangy fragrance. Its richness is in its high fatty acids content.

This oil is used both medicinally and for its cosmetic properties. Packed with anti-oxidants as well as punicic and ellagic acids, all of which are well-known and effective anti-ageing agents.

Pomegranate seed oil is also known to be both anti-inflammatory and anti-microbial and this makes it a useful oil for treating such conditions as dandruff, psoriasis and other skin and scalp conditions that may arise from irritants or as allergies to pollutants in the environment.

This oil is costly because even a small quantity of the oil requires a large amount of fruit pulp to produce, but a few drops of the oil, added to a carrier oil such as olive oil, safflower or coconut, will enhance the action of the base oil and make the concentrated essence of Pomegranate go much further.

This is a hair oil that absorbs easily and has great moisturizing properties. It adds lustre and sheen together with exceptional nutrient value.

Pomegranate seed oil is a stable oil with a respectable shelf life of two years.

*****

Peppermint Oil

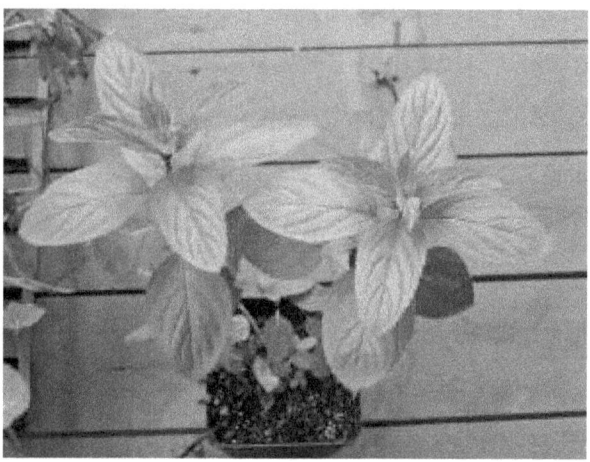

Photo Credit. JYL Cat. www.flickr.com/photos/jylcat. Creative Commons

Peppermint oil can be used on the hair. This concentrated oil has some very useful antiseptic, regenerative properties aside from being a cooling and cleansing oil.

A few drops of Peppermint added to one of the carrier oils such as Coconut, Olive or Jojoba Oil will enhance their effectiveness and action on the hair. You can also add a few drops to your shampoo and or conditioner and this will enhance its cleansing properties as well as stimulate new hair growth.

Peppermint is a crossbreed plant that originated in Europe. It is part Water Mint and part Spearmint.

Benefits for Hair.

1. The oil from the Peppermint plant has a natural balancing effect on the PHP of the scalp. It increases circulation as well as stimulating the hair follicles thereby enhancing hair growth.

2. Its anti-bacterial action helps to ease inflammation of the scalp and has a wonderfully soothing and cooling effect.

3. As a stimulant for hair growth, one can immediately feel the effects of this oil after application. A tingling sensation will spread over the scalp, enhancing circulation and stimulating blood flow to the scalp and hair roots.

4. It is also a great addition to the general health of the scalp. It is said to cure dry scalp or oily scalp by balancing the natural hair oils.

5. It will effectively treat dandruff and is also effective in getting rid of headlice... a much safer and nontoxic option than the chemical-laced lice treatments widely used these days.

This oil is a great addition to one's over-all hair care.

*****

Red Palm Oil

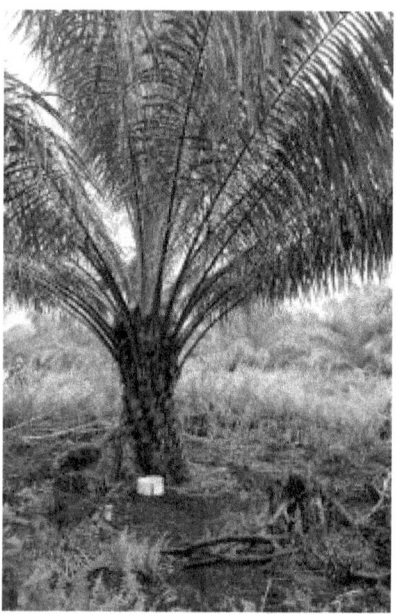

Photo Credit. CIFOR. www.flickr.com/photos/cifor. Creative Commons

Red Palm oil is obtained from the fruit of the oil palm tree. It is a reddish colour and this is said to be due to its high beta-carotene content. Red Palm oil is not to be confused with Palm Kernel oil. Red Palm oil is derived from the mesocarp of the Red Palm Fruit, whereas Palm Kernel oil is derived from the kernels of the Palm tree.

It has a long and illustrious history and has been used and appreciated since at least the time of the Egyptians.

Properties. Palm Kernel oil contains saturated fatty acids up to 89% and does not contain anything like the nutritional value of the Red Palm oil, which in turn contains mainly palmitic and oleic acids which are so beneficial for hair and skincare. Giving the Palm tree its distinctive reddish tone is the high content of carotenes, namely beta-carotene and lycopene. The oil is also rich in anti-oxidants and the Vitamin E, in particular, the tocotrienols.

Just so we get this point very clear because it is important, **Red Palm Oil**, unlike Palm Kernel oil, **is one of the most nutrient-rich foods on the planet!** In its virgin and organic form, it is an oil par none.

Benefits for Hair.

1. An effective moisturizer and conditioner for hair.

2. An emollient.

3. A richly nourishing oil.

4. Greatly assists in the regeneration and repair of damaged and weakened hair.

Shelf Life. Red Palm oil is a stable oil due to the high quantities of Vitamins A and E. If properly stored it should be usable for approximately two years.

Side Effects. Caution should be exercised where known allergies exist.

****

Rosehip Oil

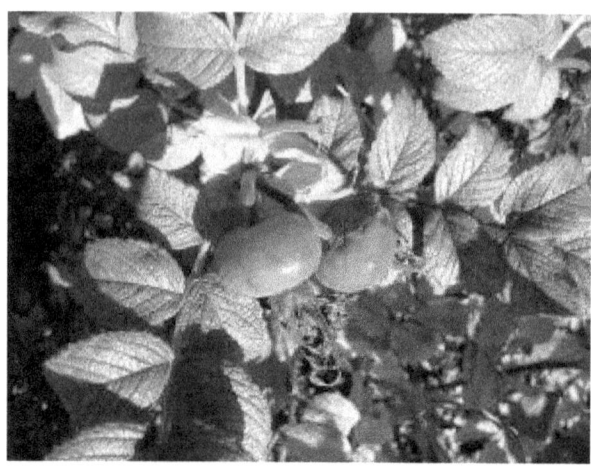

Photo Credit. Sirpale 79. www.flickr.com/photos/sirpale79. Creative Commons

Rosehip Oil is derived from the seeds of the rosebud pod of a rose bush that grows wild in the mountains of the Andes. It has a number of unique qualities as a vegetable oil and has been found to be useful in the treatment of various skin and scalp conditions.

Properties. This oil is the only known vegetable oil to contain high quantities of Vitamin A, primarily, retinol. However, it also contains high quantities of Vitamin C and the essential fatty acids of linoleic, oleic, omega 3 and omega 6.

Benefits for Hair. There are a number of benefits that come with the use of this oil as a hair care product.

1. An effective emollient and conditioner.

2. Helps to restore damaged, weakened and split hairs.

3. Is effective in the treatment of scalp disorders such as dandruff, psoriasis, and dry scaly scalp.

4. Assists in balancing the scalps natural oil production, thereby promoting and maintaining healthy hair growth.

5. Enhances the lustre, sheen, and natural hair colour.

Other Uses. It is used widely in skincare products and has been found to treat scarring, very effectively if applied regularly. It is also a great oil for use in anti-aging creams and products due to its high content of anti-oxidants.

Shelf Life. The oil is mostly produced in Chile and Argentina, where the rose bushes grow wild. It has a rather short shelf life of approximately six months and it is advised that upon opening the sealed bottle, it is best to store it in the fridge. The cold-pressed and organic version of this oil has a shorter shelf life than the processed brands, which is something to keep in mind.

Indications. As an organic and naturally grown product, this oil is not known to have toxins that can be harmful to sensitive skins, but as is always advised, care should be taken when first using the oil in order to gauge if one may have an allergic reaction, especially if known allergies are already present.

*****

Rosemary Oil

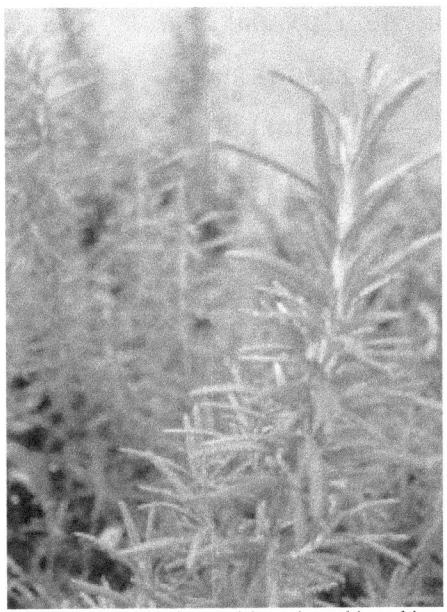

Photo Credit. Sugar Hiccup. www.flickr.com/photos/sugarhiccuphiccup. Creative Commons

Rosemary oil is rather famous as an oil that helps to promote hair growth but it also has a great fragrance, very fresh and invigorating. It is widely used throughout the Mediterranean both for its culinary taste and its healthful and medicinal properties. But this oil is not just popular in the Mediterranean countries, its reach is universal and it has a long and established history.

Benefits for Hair.

1. This oil has properties for stimulating the blood vessels when massaged regularly into the scalp.

2. It is anti-microbial. It also has antiseptic properties and is also an astringent. This makes it useful in the treatment of various scalp conditions such as psoriasis which may interfere with normal and healthy hair growth.

3. Pleasant and fresh fragrance.

4. Moisturizes and conditions the hair.

A few drops of this oil added to a carrier oil such as olive, coconut or sweet almond oils, can then be massaged into the scalp, thereby stimulating the scalp and the roots of the hair while also nourishing and moisturizing the hair shafts. It has a generally pleasing aroma and is a good 'stay in' oil.

Shelf Life. Rosemary oil has a shelf life of approximately one year.

Side Effects.

Rosemary Oil is generally thought to be a 'safe oil' however it is advised that pregnant woman or those suffering from epilepsy should avoid its use. It has also been noted that those with high blood pressure should use this oil with caution. As always those with known allergies should exercise care.

It is hard to imagine a collection of essential oils for hair without the inclusion of Rosemary oil, it has such a deeply entrenched history of use in various places around the globe.

*****

Rooibos Oil

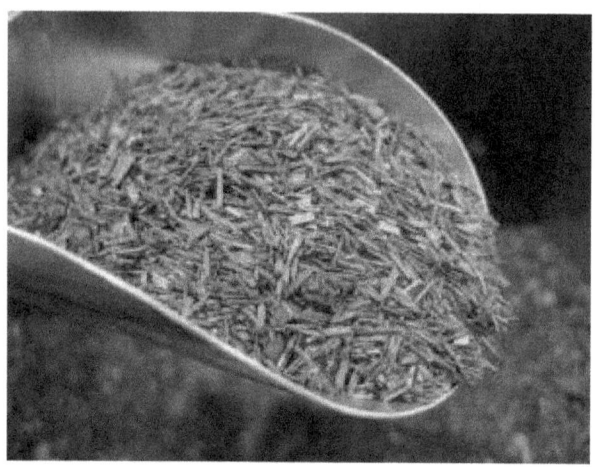

Rooibos Oil, which is derived from the African plant called Rooibos, has great restorative properties and is primarily used as a tissue oil that moisturizes and nourishes the skin.

In hair treatments, it has been found to be effective if one applies it to the hair 15 minutes before shampooing. This enables the oil to be absorbed into the hair shafts greatly assisting in moisturizing and conditioning the hair.

Although not widely known in western countries, this oil does have a long and established history on the African continent and is regarded as a valuable liniment oil and one that helps in the quick healing of scars and the restoration of normal cell tissue where there has been stretching or prior scarring has taken place.

When used on the hair it is known to have deep moisturizing effects, is quickly absorbed and adds shine and lustre to the hair and of course assists in untangling those long locks. It can be applied directly to the hair and scalp twenty minutes before shampooing.

This oil can be pricey and is not so readily available, but for those who are feeling a little extravagant and adventurous, it could well be an interesting addition to one's overall hair care plan.

*****

Soybean Oil.

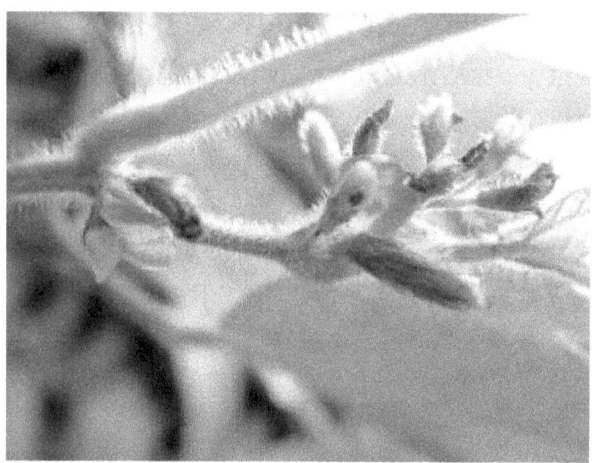

Photo Credit. Jimmy Smith. www.flickr.com/photos/jimmysmith. Creative Commons

Soybean oil and hair growth are being spoken of in the same breath more and more these days. We speak of Olive oil as an effective carrier oil for nourishing and conditioning the hair, but Soybean oil is being touted as being five times more effective. Let's investigate these claims.

Properties. This oil contains a high percentage of essential fatty acids and in particular Omega 3 and 6 fatty acids which are known to have valuable rehydrating and conditioning properties for skin and hair. The oil is also very rich in proteins. It contains mono and polyunsaturated fatty acids.

Soybean Oil and Hair Growth. The implication of increased hair growth appears to be due to Soybean oils high protein content which is easily absorbed by the hair due to the presence of long-chain fatty acids which are also prevalent in this oil. Regular application and massaging into the scalp is said to greatly improve its effectiveness.

Benefits for Hair.

1. Effective moisturizer and conditioner.

2. Rehydrates and protects the hair.

3. A highly nourishing oil.

4. Adds sheen and lustre to the hair.

5. Protects dry hair, rehydrating it.

6. Protects hair with split ends from further breaking and damage.

Shelf Life. Depending on how it is processed. A refined Soybean oil can have a shelf life of up to two years if stored correctly, but an organic brand is likely to degenerate rapidly after approximately four months due to high content levels of Omega 3 and 6 fatty acids.

Side Effects. No noted adverse side effects to the external use of this oil. It has been said, however, that it can be useful in repelling mosquitoes. If known allergies are present, caution is advised.

Shea Butter Oil

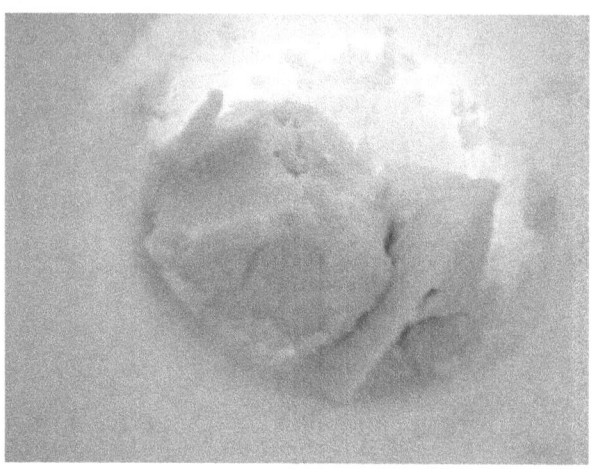

Photo Credit. Misty Kelly. www.flickr.com/photos/lilybaysoap. Creative Commons

Shea Butter Oil, which is derived from the Shea Tree, a native African plant, is loaded with fatty acids. That includes oleic, linoleic, palmitic and the list goes on. All the juicy stuff that our skin and hair crave is jam-packed into this substance.

The butter in its raw state is absorbent and non-greasy and a great repairer for damaged hair split ends and hair that just needs a bit of good old 'butter love'. This is a fabulous product and has proven its worth according to reviews and those who have been using this butter regularly. It also doesn't cost a pot of gold either! Shea butter, in its raw and unprocessed state, can be bought cheaply online via outlets such as Amazon, where it is being sold as a raw, pure and unadulterated product.

If you like to mix it with other oils this is easy to achieve and can enhance the action of the butter depending on what you use with it.

With Shea Butter, we have a multifunctional product that has a long shelf life. This is an oil that is well worthy of our attention and bound to gain as much prominence in the world of hair care as it has already deservedly gained in the realm of skincare.

Shea Butter Oil is a fractionated form of Shea Butter. This processing separates the liquid olein from the solid stearin components. The oil is often used in shampoos and conditioners and makes an excellent oil for a hot oil hair treatment.

As already mentioned, it is not a costly oil and the shelf life is between one and two years.

*****

Sea Buckthorn Oil

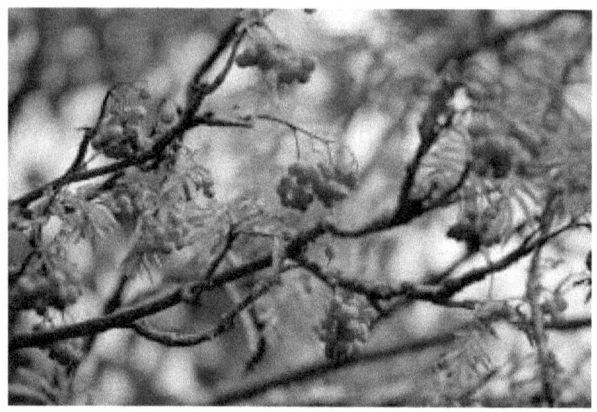

Photo Credit. Volker Moebius. www.flickr.com/photos/vmoebius. Creative Commons

Sea Buckthorn oil is derived from a thorny shrub that is cultivated mainly in China but grows abundantly throughout Asia. It thrives near water and grows in sandy soils. It has long been valued in Asian countries as a medicinal plant with a multitude of healing properties.

The medicinal benefits of this plant are in fact too numerous to mention and not required in this study but they cover anything from reducing high blood pressure to lowering cholesterol and healing stomach ulcers.

For our purposes, however, it enough to say that the oil produced from Sea Buckthorn is nutrient-rich and contains many anti-oxidants, vitamins, minerals, amino acids and fatty acids. This powerful concoction as a hair oil makes a wonderful nourishing oil and moisturizer. It is also effective in treating skin conditions and as such is useful as a scalp treatment for dandruff and other irritations that can afflict the scalp.

Sea Buckthorn oil absorbs easily and does not leave any greasy traces on the hair or skin. Because it is so nutrient-rich and also so easily assimilated into the skin and hair follicles it is an oil that is very beneficial for the hair.

It has a reasonable shelf life of one year and as we always say with the hair oils, where possible buy the cold-pressed organic brands in order to get an oil that has been processed as little as possible thereby retaining the maximum goodness and benefits.

Needless to say that Sea Buckthorn is an oil to look out for and one that is worth its weight in gold for the conditioning and health of our hair.

*****

Sesame Oil

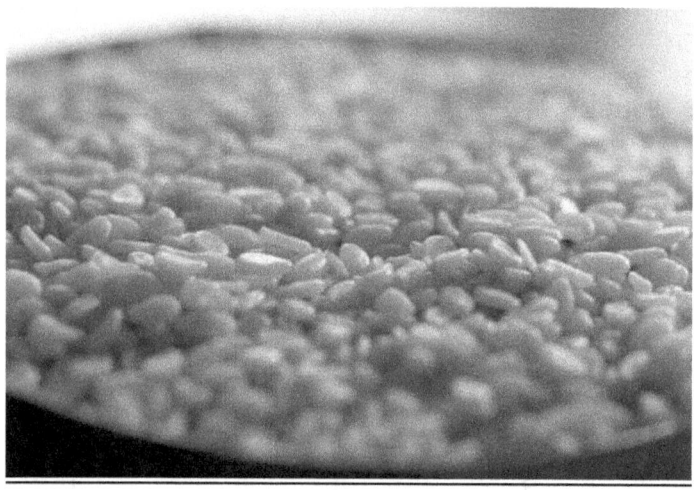

Photo Credit.Sweet Beet and Green Bean. www.flickr.com/photos/sweetbeetandgreenbean.Creative Commons

Sesame oil may well be a secret for your hair because you may not have even realized that it can be used as a hair oil and a very effective one at that.

Sesame Seeds have been around for a very long time. In fact, they have been noted to have been a part of ancient cultures in both Africa and India some thousands of years ago.

When I am in India I often come across sesame sweets and other delights for the palate made with these nutrition-packed, tasty little seeds. The oil is just as readily available in this country as the sweets and edibles are and forms a fundamental part of day-to-day life. It is used in cooking, it is used by the Brahmins in the Hindu temples for the lamps that are offered to the Gods, it is used on the skin and what is not so widely known is that it is also used on the hair.

This is one amazing oil. It is rich in fatty acids and proteins, anti-oxidants and amino acids. The list goes on...

Aside from all this nutritional value, Sesame seeds also contain many valuable medicinal qualities such as being anti-microbial, anti-fungal, anti-inflammatory and so on. These properties make it a great oil to be rubbed into the scalp for the control of dandruff, dry scaly scalp, and psoriasis.

Indian Ayurvedic medicines use this oil in many of their oil-based medicines and it plays a central part in the composition of many of their treatments, hair based and otherwise.

Look for an organic, cold-pressed Sesame oil. The shelf life of Sesame Oil can vary according to environmental conditions and the manner in which it is stored, but it's not so very long. It is advisable that the oil you purchase is within the 6 month limit of its expiry date.

Safflower Oil

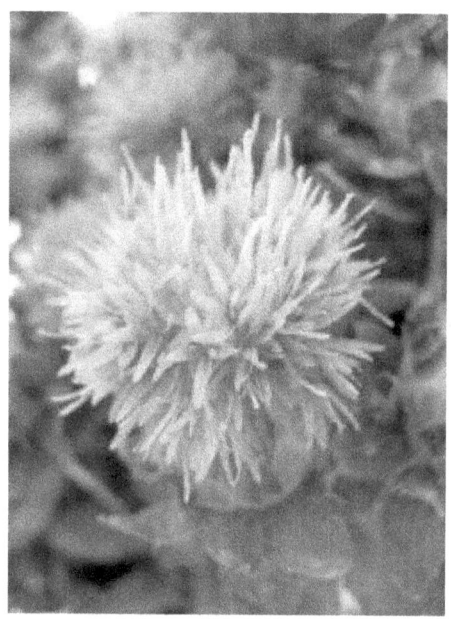

Photo Credit. GNIKRJ. www.flickr.com/photos/gnikrj . Creative Commons

Safflower Oil is usually thought of more as an oil that appears in the kitchen and not one for the bathroom cupboard. Yet here are some interesting facts about its benefits as a topical oil for both skin and hair.

Firstly the Safflower oil, not to be confused with Sunflower oil, is derived from the seeds of the Safflower plant. It is a light oil that is colourless and flavourless.

There are two types of Safflower oil, one is high in monounsaturated fatty acids, (oleic acids). The other is high in polyunsaturated fatty acids, (linoleic acids). The first oil is the one usually found in the kitchen and is used in cooking, salads etc.

Both oils have valuable moisturizing properties and are very beneficial as hair conditioners and moisturizers.

The Good News for your Hair

Safflower oil is a good choice as a carrier oil to which a few drops of essential oil can be added in order to enhance its effectiveness if used on the hair.

If this oil is massaged thoroughly into the scalp and hair regularly it will add a protective layer that shields the hair from harsh environmental changes and pollutants while moisturizing and nourishing it at the same time.

It has also been found that massaging this oil into the scalp regularly has a similar effect as a vasodilator which will dilate blood vessels in and around the hair roots, which in turn allows for better blood circulation and healthier conditions for the regrowth and overall accelerated growth of hair.

Safflower oil is cost-effective along with being widely and easily available but it is important to keep in mind that there are two types of Safflower oil. Both will have beneficial effects for your hair so where possible try to get cold-pressed Safflower oil as the pressing will have had the least effect on that valuable EFAs which our hair and skin so badly need as we get older.

Safflower oil is an all-around excellent choice as a hair oil and well worth trying out to see if this is a hair oil for you.

*****

Olive Squalane

Olive Squalane is the synthesized cousin of Olive Squalene which is naturally occurring and has been dubbed the 'natural moisturizer.' Because it is much cheaper, it is Olive Squalane that is often produced and used in cosmetic and some hair oil preparations. Many people are not aware of this difference or that there even is one in the first place.

Olive Squalene, on the other hand, is costly and has a much shorter shelf life than its cousin Olive Squalane.

Olive Squalane is a good deal cheaper and has a more stable composition which gives it a longer shelf life and therefore greater usability. What is of particular interest with this oil is its affinity with the skin. It contains a botanical lipid that closely resembles that of human skin's sebaceous cells. Because the oil is vegetable-based and not animal-based and easily assimilated by human skin of all types. It is also good and safe choice as a skin and hair moisturizer, especially if you have known allergies or are particularly sensitive.

Olive Squalane is essentially a light and stable version of olive oil. Because it is so light it is easily absorbed into the skin and hair shafts providing a high level of moisturizing and nutrient value without leaving any traces or greasiness on the skin or hair.

Here we list the benefits of Squalane in both skin and hair care.

1. It has anti-bacterial properties which make it useful to use on skin and for scalp conditions such as rashes and eczema, dandruff and psoriasis.

2. Absorbs easily, so it makes a great moisturizer.

3. Useful for rehydration and as an intensive conditioner for the skin and hair.

4. Treats chapped and cracked skin and helps to repair and regenerate damaged or weakened hair.

5. Helps to reduce wrinkles.

6. Protects hair and skin against harsh environmental pollutants and extremes of heat, cold, wind and rain.

For the hair, it is an excellent moisturizer and a slightly costly but effective carrier hair oil that does not leave the hair feeling heavy, glumpy or greasy.

If stored properly in a cool and dark place this oil has a long shelf life of approximately 25 to 28 months.

*****

Tamanu Oil

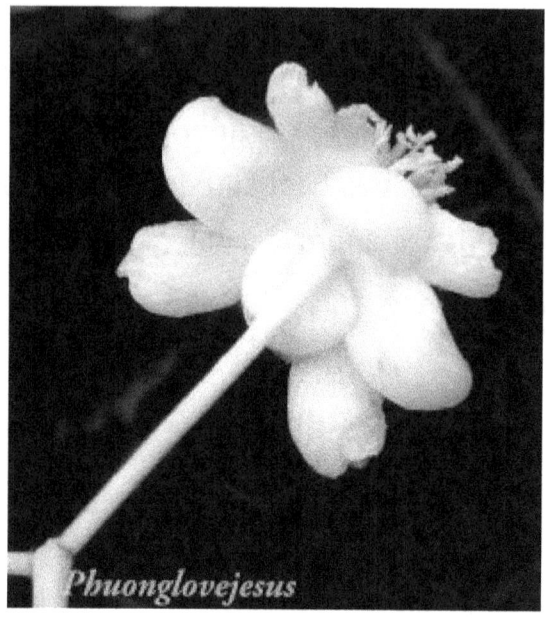

Photo Credit.Vietnam and USA Plants. www.flickr.com/photos/phuonglovejesus2782010.Creative Commons

Tamanu Oil originates in Polynesia where it is pressed from the nuts of the Ati tree. Although primarily used in skincare products, the oil of this nut is also considered highly beneficial for the hair. It has long been used in the South Pacific Islands for a wide range of purposes but has only recently been taken up by researchers from the west and is now beginning to generate some real and deserved interest.

Properties. This oil has concentrated amounts of essential fatty acids. It contains a compound known as calophyllolide (a substance that has anti-inflammatory properties. It also contains delta-tocotrienol which is a form of the Vitamin E, along with a number of other anti-oxidants.

Benefits for Hair.

1. This oil is a superior conditioner and moisturizer.

2. It has anti-microbial and anti-inflammatory and anti-viral properties which make it useful for treating scalp conditions such as psoriasis and dandruff to name a few.

3. It not only rehydrates the hair shaft but is also noted for its ability to regenerate and strengthen weakened and compromised hair.

4. Its emollient action assists in protecting the hair from harsh environmental pollutants and extremes of dry, cold and wind. In any conditions that would strip the hair of its natural moisturizers, this oil comes into its own.

5. It works well on curly and dry hair, protecting it and helping to limit this hair types natural propensity for breakage and splitting.

5. Another interesting property of Tamanu oil is its high absorption rate. It is quickly drawn into the pores of the skin

and leaves no oily traces on the surface. The same goes with its use on the hair.

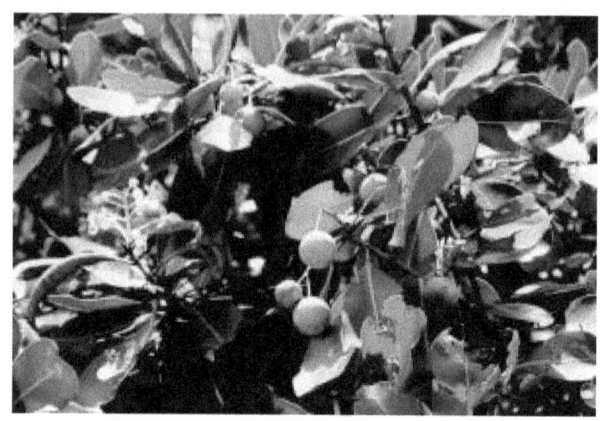

Photo Credit: Adadulokia. Creative Commons

Other Uses. It has a unique capacity to promote regeneration of skin tissue. For this reason, it has long been used by the Polynesian Islanders for everything from baby rash to skin eruptions and abrasions.

Although the Ati tree that produces the Tamanu Oil grows widely throughout South East Asia, the oil produced from its nuts is most widely used in the South Pacific.

When the fruit is harvested and once they are opened, they reveal a large white nut that appears to have no oil at all. These are then kept and dried on racks for several weeks until they turn a dark brown shade. At this stage, they are fairly dripping with oil which is then collected through a simple pressing process.

This is a rich and silky oil with very beneficial healing properties and is bound to become more widely known in the coming years.

Tamanu oil is costly and can be purchased online at various outlets and health stores.

Always check that the oil is cold-pressed in order to be sure that you are buying a product that retains the maximum amount of nutrients.

Tamanu oil has a **long shelf life** of two years or more if correctly stored.

Indications. There is an indication that this oil could cause some who are allergic or who have skin sensitivity to have an adverse reaction so I would advise some caution if there are known allergies present. More studies need to be done to fully determine the safety aspects of using this oil.

*****

Tea Tree Oil

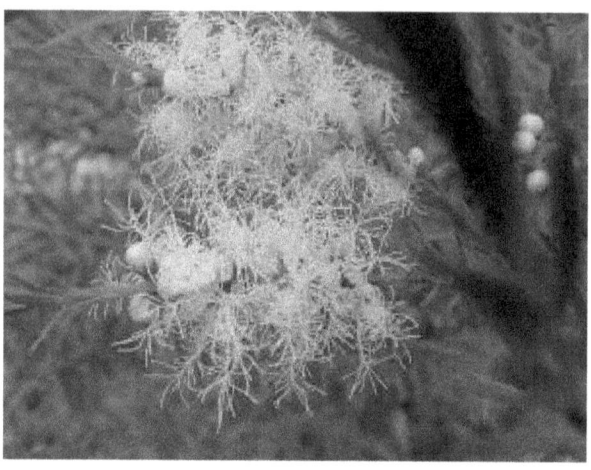

Photo Credit. Arthur Chapman. www.flickr.com/photos/arthur_chapman. Creative Commons

Tea Tree Oil is a concentrated or essential oil that is highly potent and is multifunctional. It has many benefits and uses in hair care. This Australian native gives an oil that is colourless but has a strong pungent odour.

The oil has powerful antiseptic properties as well as being an effective anti-fungal.

This is seriously not an oil to take internally. **Tea Tree oil is for external use only and,** although I have used Tea Tree oil in its undiluted state for numerous small ailments, including the treatment of Dandruff, I would suggest that one should dilute the oil with a carrier oil such as olive, coconut or jojoba before applying it. This way you will be not be exposing yourself to too much trouble should there be a reaction.

Word has been going around lately that Tea Tree oil promotes hair growth. This would make sense because it treats scalp conditions very efficiently as I know from first-hand use of this oil over a period of many years.

It works by unclogging the pores and hair follicles, balancing the scalp's natural oils and treating underlying scalp conditions with its powerful anti-fungal and anti-microbial properties. However, it should be kept in mind, that whether this oil is helpful in treating hair loss and promoting hair growth will depend on the underlying causes.

Some caution should be used when applying Tea Tree oil. NEVER use it in an undiluted form in large amounts on the skin and as we already mentioned above,

DO NOT take this oil internally.

The Shelf life of Tea Tree Oil is approximately two to three years depending on how it is stored.

In summary, there is no doubt that is this a useful and important essential oil with many benefits for the treatment of scalp conditions. It is an essential oil that you can experiment with. For instance, I add a few drops of Tea Tree and Peppermint oil to a carrier oil such as coconut and find this very effective in treating flaky scalp and dandruff. There are many other useful combinations that greatly relieve annoying scalp conditions.

*****

Ungurahua Oil

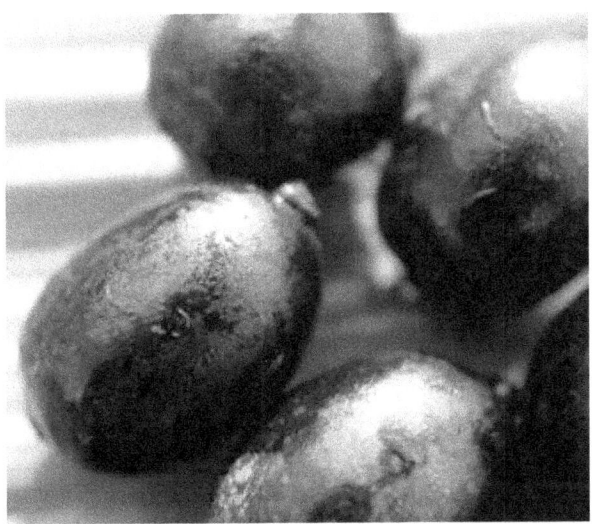

Ungurahua Oil is an exotic oil that hails from the tropical rainforests of Columbia. It is extracted from the mesocarp or middle layer of the fruit of the Seje Palm which is a native of Colombian forests.

This oil is yellowish, green in colour and transparent. It is odourless and quite similar in appearance and composition to that of Olive oil.

Known for its properties as a great fortifier of weak and damaged hair, it is said to regenerate and nourish both scalp and hair follicles.

Women from the Quechua-Shuar tribes have been using this oil for countless generations because of its wonderful restorative properties and its capacity to make the hair feel and look thicker.

It has a high absorption capacity and is quickly and easily assimilated into the hair shaft, deeply penetrating the hair's cortex and thereby strengthening it while also restoring the hair shafts natural oil balance.

It has a uniquely high quantity of unsaturated fatty acids, in particular, that of Omega 9. It is a great choice for skin and hair care products and has been used by the locals of Columbia for many generations as a hair care tonic and revitalizer which promotes hair growth. Some salons are also claiming that it enhances and maintains the natural colour and lustre of the hair.

It is an excellent emollient and has high nutritive content that absorbs quickly and without leaving greasy traces on the hair and skin.

This oil is also being marketed currently under the name of Rahua Oil. It has a long shelf life of approximately eighteen months if stored properly.

Vitamin E Oil

Vitamin E Oil benefits for hair have long been known and appreciated.

According to Wikipedia, Vitamin E Oil "refers to a group of eight fat-soluble compounds that include both tocopherols and tocotrienols.[1] Of the many different forms of vitamin E, γ-tocopherol is the most common in the North American diet.[2] γ-Tocopherol can be found in corn oil, soybean oil, margarine, and dressings.[3][4] In the North American diet, α-tocopherol, the most biologically active form of vitamin E, is the second-most common form of vitamin E. This variant can be found most abundantly in wheat germ oil, sunflower, and safflower oils.[4][5] As a fat-soluble antioxidant, it stops the production of reactive oxygen species formed when fat undergoes oxidation."

Hopefully, the above quotation will give the reader an idea of the origins of Vitamin E oil. I am still a little puzzled over how a concentrated extract of Vitamin E would be generated.

It does appear however that the carrier oils Wheat Germ, and Safflower, which we already know are great for use as base hair oils, also contain a generous amount of this valuable vitamin. I generally prefer to use a natural vitamin source, but as this is a sought-after oil for hair I decided to add a post on it for those interested.

Those who advocate the use of this oil claim that it does wonders for hair growth and as such can treat all manner of scalp and hair conditions. Any oil that has properties that are of benefit in skin and scalp conditions will b useful when it comes to hair regeneration and stimulating follicle growth.

The shelf life of this oil can vary, from between one and three years, but this mostly depends on how it is stored. If refrigerated and kept in a dark and cool place, this will extend its usefulness.

*****

Wheatgerm Oil

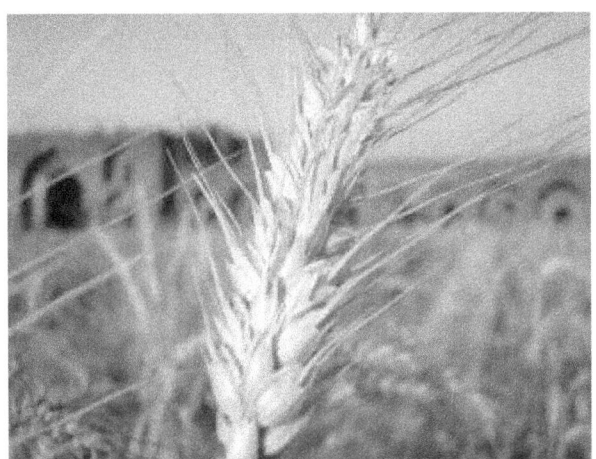

Photo Credit. Souvikdg. www.flickr.com/photos/souvikdg. Creative Commons

Wheat Germ Oil, although normally taken internally, can also be used topically and is an excellent moisturizer for skin and hair.

Properties. Wheat Germ oil contains many long-chain fatty acids which make it a good choice as an emollient. It has an estimated 75% polyunsaturated fatty acid content. The vitamins E and A are also plentiful in this oil and add greatly to its nutritive value as well as enhancing its effectiveness as a moisturizer. Wheat Germ oil is also high in vitamins D and the B complex as well as being a concentrated source of protein. So as you can see, this oil can bestow many nutritive benefits that are essential for both skin and hair.

Benefits for Hair.

1. An excellent emollient and moisturizer.

2. Highly nutritive for the hair shaft and skin and easily absorbed by both.

3. Helps to restore and protect damaged and dry hair.

4. Promotes hair growth and re-growth by stimulating new cell growth and tissue formation.

5. Is an effective conditioner and helps to soften the hair.

Other Uses.

1. This oil is known to be effective in lowering the lipid count in those with high cholesterol.

2. Because it contains a high level of Vitamin E it also bestows all the health benefits of that vitamin, such as assisting those with heart conditions.

3. The oil is a natural anti-oxidant.

4. An important nutritional oil.

5. Assists in relieving constipation.

What to Look Out For. When purchasing this oil, go for a cold-pressed organic oil brand. The consistency of this oil is thick and has a dark amber colour with a slightly nutty odour. It has a fairly limited shelf life of between 6 to 8 months and once opened it would be advisable to refrigerate it in order to maximize its nutrients and usefulness.

Indications. If you have any known wheat or gluten allergies it would be best to avoid using this oil. Aside from this, there are no other known indications and the oil is very safe to use.

*****

Watermelon Seed Oil

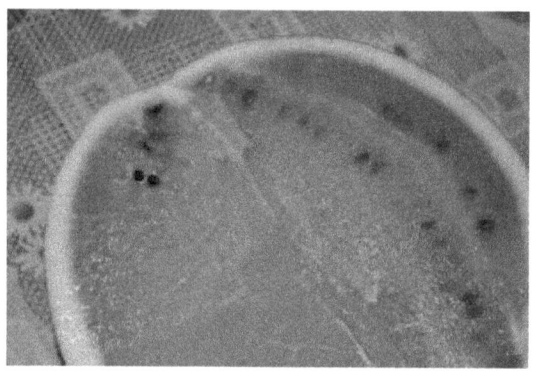

Photo Credit:Whologwhy. www.flickr.com/photos/hulagway . Creative Commons

Watermelon seed oil has long been used on the African continent where it is known by the names of Kalahari oil and Ootanga oil. The Kalahari is an extreme environment where heat, cold and dry are prevalent. Watermelon seed oil has long been used by the Bushmen to protect their hair and skin from the harsh environmental conditions.

Properties. This is a light oil with potent moisturizing properties and a high content of essential fatty acids, namely omega 9 and omega 6.

Benefits for Hair.

1. It absorbs into the skin and hair quickly and completely not clogging the pore or hair follicles as mineral oil do.

2. This oil protects the hair from harsh extremes of dry and cold, heat and wind.

3. It is also a restorative not only rehydrating but enabling the hair to retain its moisture.

4. It nourishes the hair and skin with its numerous fatty acids and vitamins.

5. It is not a greasy oil and has excellent emollient properties.

6. It helps to dissolve sebum build-up.

Shelf Life. This is a stable oil with a long shelf life due to its high concentration of EFAs and vitamins.

Indications. The oil is not taken for internal use and as an external oil, it is nontoxic and not known to cause any adverse reactions. However, as with all the oils, where allergies are present and known caution should be exercised.

Ximenia Oil

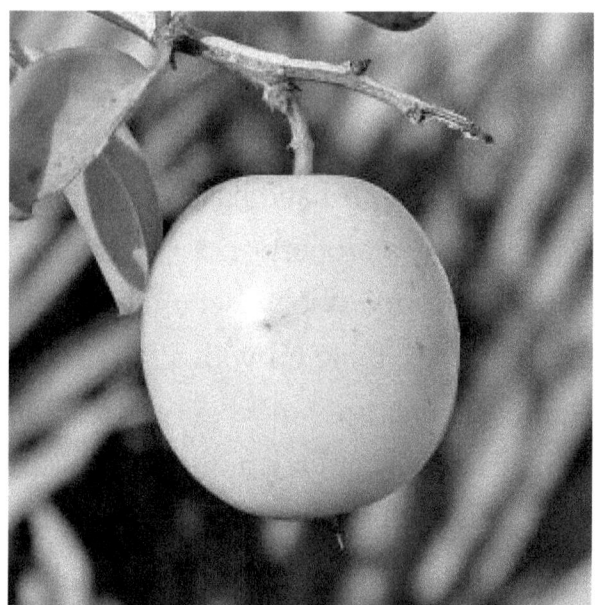

Photo Credit.Bob in Swamp. www.flickr.com/photos/pondapple. Creative Commons

Ximenia Oil is derived from a small native tree that grows abundantly in high woodlands throughout the southern areas of Africa where it is referred to locally as Wild Plum.

The oil is extracted from the kernels of the fruit of the Ximenia Tree which yields a rich oil that contains high levels of monounsaturated fatty acids which has important moisturizing properties for both skin and hair.

Properties. Ximenia oil has a 92% unsaturated fatty acid profile. Very impressive! It also contains saturated and long-chain fatty acids. It contains proteins and a high percentage of Vitamin C in the mature fruit stage of some 25%.

Benefits for Hair.
1. This is a highly nourishing conditioner.
2. It has also been shown to enhance circulation of the blood and it is suggested that regular massaging of the oil into the skin and the scalp at the base of the hair roots will stimulate hair growth and rejuvenate the scalp helping it to rebalance in natural oils.
3. An emollient oil that protects from extremes in environmental conditions.
4. This is a rehydrating oil that seals in its moisture.
5. It has a highly nourishing profile and bestows regenerative benefits for dry and damaged hair and skin.
6. Contains natural anti-inflammatory properties that make it useful in conditions of dandruff and psoriasis.
7. Has natural anti-microbial and anti-fungal properties which augment its usefulness in the treatment of scalp problems.

Shelf Life. This is a stable oil with a long shelf life of approximately two years.

Side Effects. None have been noted, however, caution should be exercised where known allergies exist.

*****

Ylang Ylang Oil

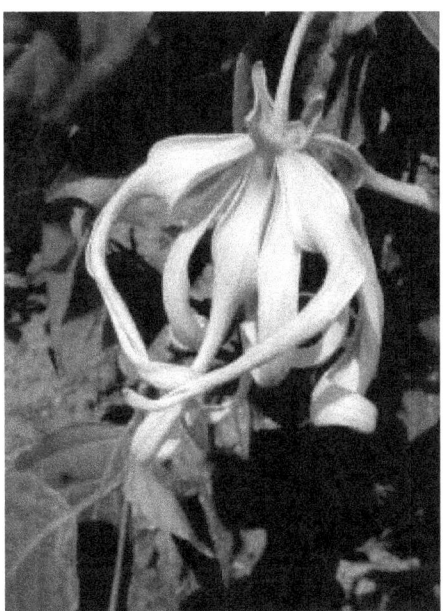

Photo Credit. Adaduitokla.
www.flickr.com/photos/adaduitokla. Creative Common

Ylang Ylang Oil is derived from the Ylang Ylang tree or the Cananga tree as it is also known. It is a native of Indonesia and highly valued for its perfume.

Benefits for Hair.

1. Helps in balancing the scalp's sebum production, thereby normalizing the over or underproduction of scalp secretions.

2. Stimulates hair growth.

3. Soothing.

Side Effects. Ylang Ylang oil has been noted to cause headaches in some people with first use.

*****

5. Indian Hair Oils

There are so many Indian Hair Oils on the market that I could easily fill a volume just going through them all. However, that is not possible at the moment so I have only included a few of the more famous and popular oils that are used, not only in India but also now increasingly abroad in Western countries.

As I am always testing out new ones I will continue to add the best of them to this section in order to keep you all updated.

India, as you may be aware, has a long association with the use and preparation of Hair Oils, many of which are as simple as Coconut oil, but others are a complex and careful mix of various herbs and potions all geared to addressing specific problems to do with hair care and health.

Amla Oil

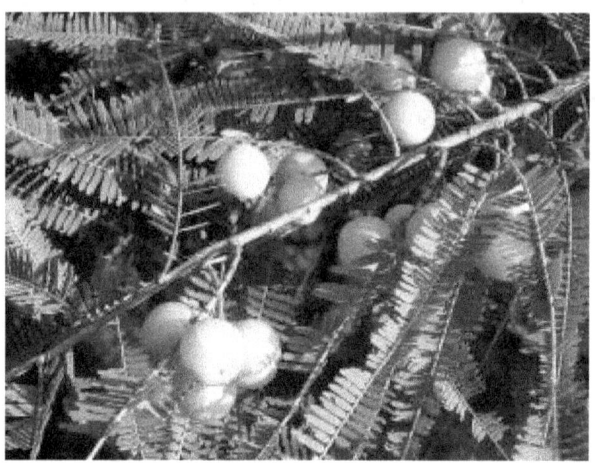

Photo Credit. Lalithamba. www.flickr.com/photos/45835639@N04. Creative Commons

Amla hair oil has been used by generations of Indian men and women to protect and nourish their and their children's hair. This oil has a long history. It is based on the old Indian medical Ayurvedic traditions which began at the time of the Vedas.

It is said to have a 'cooling' effect and is often applied just after washing the hair in order to condition and add a lustre to the hair. Aside from this, however, it is known to have a number of other important hair benefits. It helps to prevent hair greying as well as hair loss and is also said to treat dry and itchy scalp.

It contains a number of essential fatty acids that are believed to strengthen hair follicles and have a deep conditioning effect on the hair. Along with these fatty acids, it also contains various flavonoids, polyphenols, vitamins, and minerals.

One of the causes of hair breakage and split ends has been found to be Vitamin C deficiency and Amla, which is one of the most Vitamin C rich fruits on the planet, goes a long way to addressing this problem by naturally supplementing the normal supply.

The process by which it is made involves the immersion of the dried amla fruit in oil. Traditionally the oil chosen as a carrier for Amla is either coconut or sesame oil, both of which are readily available in India. This process can take a number of days to complete as the fruit needs to be immersed for a specific period of time.

Amla Oil is easily available in shops that specialize in Indian products. One should, however, be aware that it does have a rather strong and pungent smell which might detract somewhat from its use as a 'leave on' conditioner.

It is so widely used on the subcontinent that there must be some basis in fact for its long popularity. I have used itself myself at different periods and found it to be a great conditioner and very suitable as a medium hair oil. It would be too heavy for light hair, but medium to thick hair can benefit greatly from regular application.

*****

Brahmi Oil

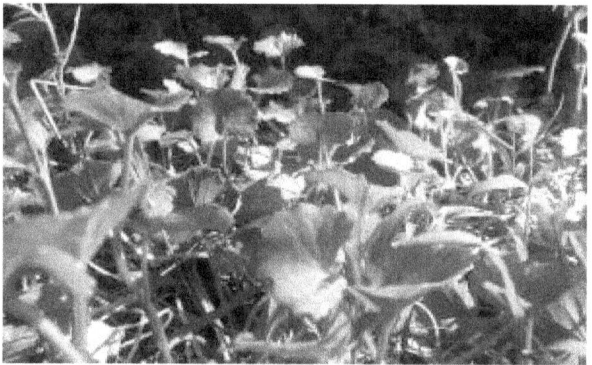

Brahmi Oil was developed by Ayurveda as a treatment for hair and scalp conditions, such as dandruff, psoriasis, dry, brittle hair, premature greying and hair fall. However, Brahmi is primarily known for its memory-enhancing capacities.
Brahmi Oil is a composite of Brahmi powder and Sesame oil. Brahmi is also known by the name of Indian Pennywort and has a long and much-respected history on the sub-continent of India. These days, however, this oil is also becoming popular in the west.

The oil is rich in antioxidants which nourish and revitalize the hair as well as calming the nervous system. A nervous system that is at ease can then be readily bought back into balance, an important starting point for natural and holistic healing.

Massaging this oil into the hair roots and scalp on a regular basis will have a number of benefits. It not only stimulates the hair follicles, thus promoting hair growth, but it also treats scalp conditions such as psoriasis, dandruff, dry and flaky scalp.

Aside from those considerable benefits it will also moisturize and condition the hair while nourishing it with its many anti-oxidants.

The use of a little of this oil, which can be massaged into the scalp just before bed, is also said to treat insomnia and assist in relaxing and de-stressing.

This oil is a composite of Brahmi Powder steeped in Sesame Oil. It has a shelf life approximately one year.

*****

Mira Oil

It is interesting to note just how much misinformation there is about Mira Oil. Therefore, we will endeavour to put this right by offering you the results of some careful research.

Mira Oil originated in India many thousands of years ago. It is a natural non-toxic blend of oils that was first put together by India's Ayurvedic Doctors following their carefully guarded and time-proven methods of preparation.

It is known to be an effective hair tonic and one that contains no harmful chemicals or unpleasant side effects. It is a great 'replenisher' restoring hair that has been overworked and damaged by styling and dying or the harsh environmental factors that can dry out and damage the hair.

Over the centuries, the preparation of this oil was kept secret and generally only royalty or the very wealthy benefited from its use. It is a blend of some 13 natural oils and herbs a number of which are common and well known such as Coconut oil, Indian Sunflower, Henna etc. These ingredients are blended together with a well known Ayurvedic herb known as Brahmi. This is a perennial creeper that grows mainly in the north of India and is well known for its blending qualities and powerful action on memory enhancement and brain function. This particular herb has been used in Ayurvedic medicines for many, many centuries and has proven its effectiveness against various ailments, namely those connected with the head.

All of the ingredients in Mira oil have been carefully selected for their powerful hair nourishing, conditioning, toning effects. Certain of the herbs stimulate the scalp and invigorate the hair follicles thereby promoting hair growth. These oils and herbs, when correctly combined and prepared have an overall effect on the hair that appears to be quite stunning.

When used regularly this oil is touted to be responsible for 3 to 4 inches of hair growth a month! But there is one important factor to keep in mind. Originating, as it does, from the ancient Ayurvedic traditions of India, which encourage a holistic healing approach, there is more to this amazing result than simply applying the oil. Environmental and lifestyle factors must also be taken into consideration, along with diet and exercise. If all these factors are carefully managed and combined then the effectiveness of this oil is sure to be greatly enhanced.

This is not a cheap hair oil, you will pay good money for it and therefore it is important to be careful as to the quality of the product that you are purchasing. A verified South Indian Aryuvedic company would be a good bet when looking into product brands with reliable quality and affordable prices.

*****

Trichup Oil

I came to know about Trichup hair oil when I was staying in the South of India. I had asked one of my Indian women friends which hair oil they preferred. Lata has gorgeous long, black hair that is waist length. She immediately said the word 'Trichup Oil,' until then, I had never even heard of this particular brand.

However, one day when I was walking past an Ayurvedic shop in the town, I remembered her words and dropped into the store to ask them. Sure enough, they had a few varieties of this oil but the brand on the photo seemed to be the one most people trust.

It is a little pricey for an Indian hair oil but cheap when compared to Western hair oils and considering the ingredients, all excellent hair treatment herbs and oils with a guarantee of purity and correct processing, then it instils some confidence. I went ahead and bought a bottle.

I have been using it off and on ever since and found this oil to be very helpful for my hair. In the first place, it completely eliminates the frizz and in the second it makes it very easy to manage and without a lot of the scalp irritation that can often come with some of the hair oils.

According to the Trichup company; '*Trichup Oil is enriched with the natural goodness of Bhringraj, Amalaki, Neem, Gunja and other hair rejuvenating herbs which are processed in high-quality Sesame and Coconut oil. Sesame oil is a good source of hair nutrients like Vitamin A, E and skin-friendly fatty acids whereas Coconut oil is one of the best soothing and protection oils for hair.*'

If you have time to check out my posts on Neem, Coconut and Sesame Oils you will see that all of these have important benefits for hair, while the other herbal ingredients are well known Indian Ayurvedic herbs with useful properties for hair care.

Results are best gauged by regular treatment.

Again, according to Trichup, some of the benefits of this oil include;

"*Improves blood circulation to the scalp tissues and hair follicles.*

Revitalizes hair gives its natural bounce and lustre.

Controls hair fall and induces fresh growth.

Prevents hair discolouration by stimulating hair melanin content thus reduces premature greying."

If you are interested in trying out different Indian hair oils, this is a good place to start. Trichup Oil has arisen from a long and ancient tradition and has been tried and tested by many, many people on the subcontinent. It is also not too hard on the pocket and has a long shelf of supposedly three years.

*****

About the Author

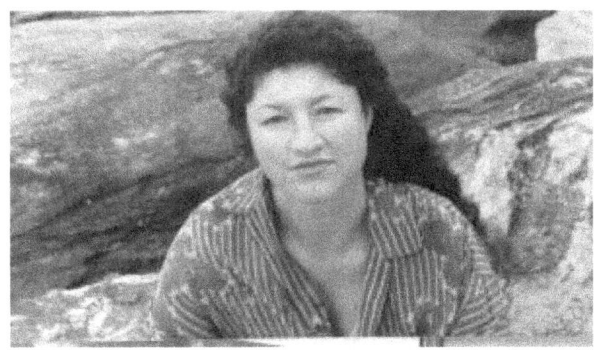

My journey into the world of 'hair oils' began at the tender age of 13 years! I was born with thick, curly, dry and unruly hair which my mother always insisted on cutting.

This set me up early for a spot of 'rebellion' from which, until this day, I have never quite outgrown. As soon as I reached puberty I refused to have my tresses lopped off. As a result, I quickly found myself with an unwieldy mop of hair. Fortunately, I was able to discover that oil could be very helpful in taming the tangle and flattening the frizz.

Thus began my 'hair oil adventures.'

Back in the 1970 s 80 s and even 90 s! there was very little in the way of Hair Care Oil-based products available for sale on the market in New Zealand and Australia where I grew up. If I wandered into the grocery store or the local chemist all I could ever find was Bryl Cream for men. A rather greasy paste that did not entice me even remotely, to plaster on my curly locks.

So I put together my own hair oils, using an intuitive mix of almond oil as a base and rosemary and other essential oils as active ingredients. This worked wonders.

Later when I moved to Australia I discovered something called 'Californian Poppy Oil.' It was readily available in the local chemists and as I was very busy with my studies during those years, I took to using that instead of my homemade concoctions. It had a rather strong fragrance and I suspect now that it may have contained at least a little mineral oil, which, instead of acting as a conditioner actually clogs up the hair follicles and prevents absorption, but nevertheless, it accompanied me through most of my twenties until the late 1980 s when I began to live in India for extended periods of time.

I assume that people are aware that India is probably the 'Hair Oil Mecca of Asia', if not the world. I felt instantly in my element. Having grown up with very little in the way of hair oiling options, I soon found myself bowled over by the sheer volume and choice of hair oils that are readily available on the sub-continent. At least when it comes to oily hair potions, creams and things for plastering on the hair.

Walk into any shop, be it a bidi walla's shop on any street corner, and you could very likely come across at least one brand of hair oil... Bliss!

Since arriving in India some few decades ago I have worked my way through just about every kind of hair oil that I could get my hands on, and there are some pretty wild and wacky ones available too I can assure you, some real yogi dread-lock potions!

I have included a few articles on Indian Hair Oils that I found to be most useful over the years and of course I have made available comprehensive information on just about every kind of Hair Oil I have ever been able to discover with the hope that those who read this book will find a detailed list and enough information to be able to make the Hair Oil choices that will be most appropriate for them.

I hope you will find the information offered here useful and that it will guide you towards making good decisions in your choice of hair oils. For each person, there might be a period of trial and error until you find exactly the right oil to suit your particular hair care needs, and it may not be the most costly oil that will be of greatest benefit to you, but then, finding this out for ourselves is all part of the adventure and I hope that Handbook of Hair Oils will give you the inspiration to delve further.

*****

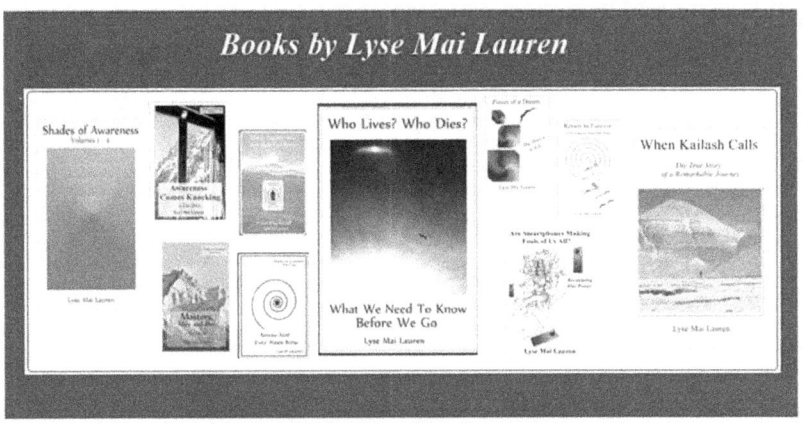

Series Shades of Awareness

Vol.1, Awareness Comes Knocking

Vol.2, Tibetan Masters and Other True Stories

Vol.3, Masters, Mice and Men

Vol.4, Never Not Eve Here Now

Who Lives, Who Dies?

hat We Need to Know Before We Go

Pieces of a Dream

Return to Forever

Are Smartphones Making Fools of us All?

When Kailash Calls

*****

Connect with me on the Website

Handbook of Hair Oils